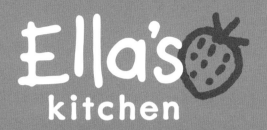

Ella's kitchen

the first foods book

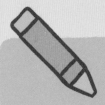

For all the babies born this year.
Eat well, grow strong — for this world is yours.

First published in Great Britain in 2015 by Hamlyn, an imprint of Octopus Publishing Group Ltd, Carmelite House, 50 Victoria Embankment, London EC4Y 0DZ
www.octopusbooks.co.uk

An Hachette UK Company
www.hachette.co.uk

This revised edition published in 2025

Distributed in the US by Hachette Book Group, 1290 Avenue of the Americas, 4th and 5th Floors, New York, NY 10104

Distributed in Canada by Canadian Manda Group, 664 Annette St, Toronto, Ontario, Canada M6S 2C8

ISBN 978-0-600-63757-8

A CIP catalogue record for this book is available from the British Library.

Printed and bound in China.

10 9 8 7 6 5 4 3 2 1

MIX
Paper | Supporting responsible forestry
FSC® C008047

Created by Ella's Kitchen
Editorial Director: Natalie Bradley
Art Director: Juliette Norsworthy
Senior Editor: Leanne Bryan
Recipe Developer: Nicola Graimes
Art direction, design + styling: Anita Mangan
Design: Billy Odell

Photographer: Jonathan Cherry
Food Stylist: Natalie Thomson
Props Stylist: Jennifer Haslam
Copy Editor: Clare Churly
Design Assistant: Ella McLean
Production Manager: Caroline Alberti

Disclaimer Check with a healthcare professional before starting weaning if your child has a family history of food allergies, asthma, eczema or other allergies. Check all packaging for allergy advice and use clean surfaces and utensils to avoid allergens sneaking into your cooking. Never give whole nuts to children under the age of 5 years in case of choking. Some recipes contain honey. It is advised not to feed honey to children under 12 months old. Every care should be taken when cooking with and for children. Neither the author nor the publisher can accept any liability for any consequences arising from the use of this book, or the information contained herein.

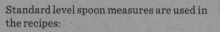

publisher's notes

Standard level spoon measures are used in the recipes:

1 tablespoon = one 15 ml spoon

1 teaspoon = one 5 ml spoon

1 ice cube = one 15 ml spoon

Both metric and imperial measurements are given for the recipes. Use one set of measurements only, not a mixture of both.

Ovens should be preheated to the specified temperature. For a fan-assisted oven, follow the manufacturer's instructions to adjust the cooking time and temperature.

Medium-sized ingredients and pans and medium-strength cheese have been used throughout unless otherwise specified. Herbs are fresh unless otherwise specified. Use low-salt stock, and avoid adding salt to recipes.

Freezing and storage

Freeze food in a freezer set at -18°C (0°F).

See pages 26 and 27 for further storage and freezing information.

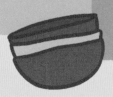

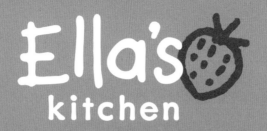

Ella's kitchen

the first foods book

the purple one

130 yummy recipes
from weaning to the big table

hamlyn

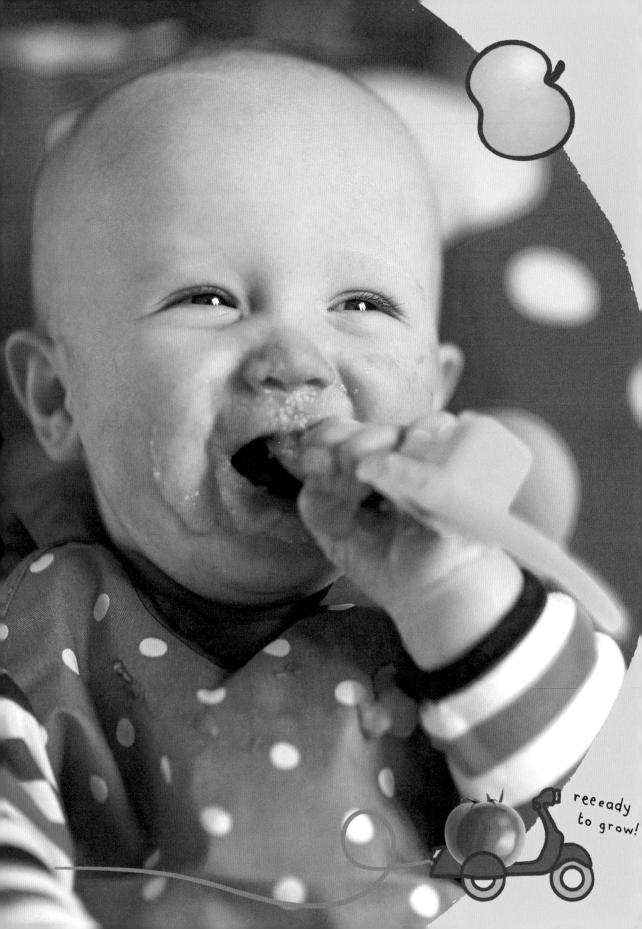

reeeady
to grow!

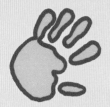

contents

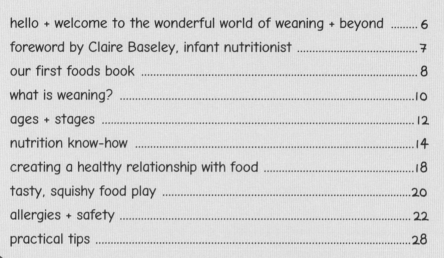

scrummy recipes!

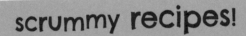

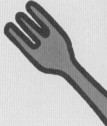
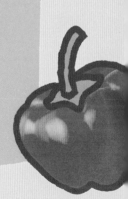
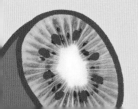

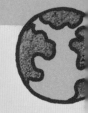

hello + welcome to the
wonderful world
of weaning + beyond

Weaning can be one of the most enjoyable but also one of the most frustrating + stressful times for both grown-ups + children. In the end, only you know what works for you + your baby. The most important thing to remember is that weaning is easiest when it's fun for little ones. When they get to play, explore + have fun with food using all their senses they become more willing to try new things and are more likely to develop a lifelong love of food.

This book joins you at the very beginning of your baby's foodie journey. It puts you in charge, gives you choices and, through its tips + advice, aims to help you develop the confidence to follow your instinct.

The whole Ella's Kitchen team has been involved in creating *The First Foods Book*, offering tips, advice + recipes. We hope you enjoy every second of using it as much as we have enjoyed creating it.

Keep smiling!

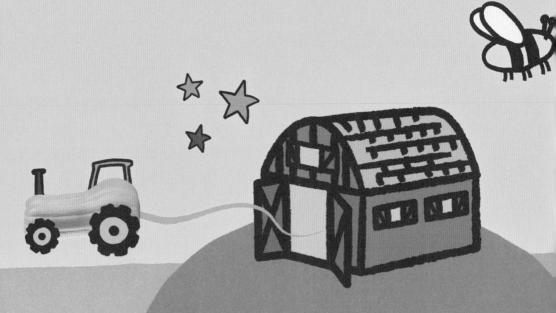

foreword by Claire Baseley,
infant nutritionist

I've worked with Ella's Kitchen for 11 years and in that time
I've been lucky enough to win an award for the good work
I do on feeding little ones.

I've met lots and lots of babies and their parents and carers
over the years. Plenty of you tell me that you find weaning
quite stressful but at the same time, you want to make it
a really fun experience for your little ones.

Some of the questions I'm asked the most frequently
are: Am I giving my baby enough to eat? What about
choking? And how do I introduce allergens, textures
or finger foods?

In this book, we've answered all of those questions
and more. But most importantly, we've shared
how you can make weaning a fun, tasty, sensory
adventure that will help your little one establish a
healthy relationship with food and take the stress
out of mealtimes.

My top tips for creating good eating habits that can last
into childhood and beyond include repeatedly offering a
variety of yummy veggies early on and throughout weaning,
letting your little one experience food with all of their
senses, and enjoying meals together as often as you can.

Above all, when it comes to eating, have lots of fun!

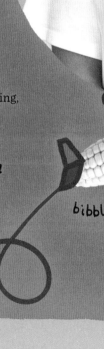

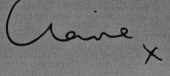

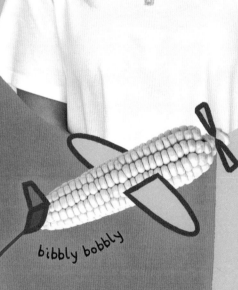

bibbly bobbly

7

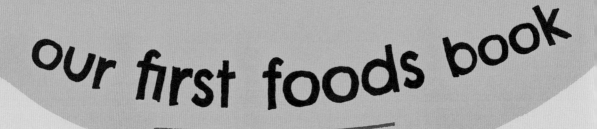

our first foods book

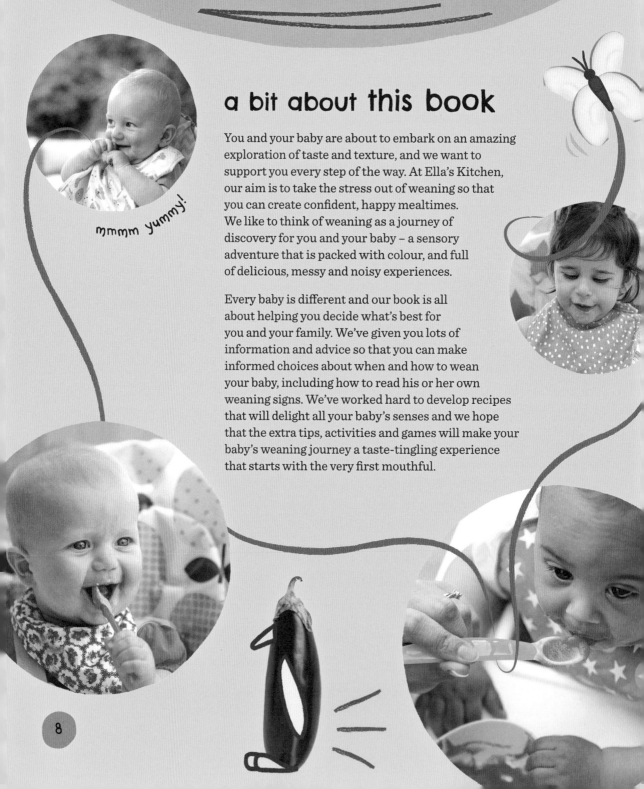

mmmm yummy!

a bit about this book

You and your baby are about to embark on an amazing exploration of taste and texture, and we want to support you every step of the way. At Ella's Kitchen, our aim is to take the stress out of weaning so that you can create confident, happy mealtimes. We like to think of weaning as a journey of discovery for you and your baby – a sensory adventure that is packed with colour, and full of delicious, messy and noisy experiences.

Every baby is different and our book is all about helping you decide what's best for you and your family. We've given you lots of information and advice so that you can make informed choices about when and how to wean your baby, including how to read his or her own weaning signs. We've worked hard to develop recipes that will delight all your baby's senses and we hope that the extra tips, activities and games will make your baby's weaning journey a taste-tingling experience that starts with the very first mouthful.

meet the experts

We've worked closely with a number of experts to make sure our recipes are as good for your baby as possible. Here are our recipe superstars:

 Claire Baseley is an Infant Nutritionist. She's helped us make sure all our ingredients are really good for tiny tummies and growing bodies.

 Nicola Graimes is an award-winning Cookery Author, specializing in children's nutrition. She's helped us write all the book's delicious recipes.

 Dr Carmel Houston-Price is a Developmental Psychologist who works with us to understand the role of the five senses in the way a baby develops healthy attitudes towards food.

 Sally Luckraft is our Food Developer. She makes all Ella's yummy new stuff. She's helped make sure our recipes will make little taste buds tingle.

key to icons

At the top of every recipe, you'll find a combination of the following symbols to help make the job of weaning your baby as easy as can be.

 How many teaspoons the recipe makes

 How many ice cubes the recipe makes

 How many pieces the recipe makes

 How many little ones the recipe serves

 How many adults and little ones this family recipe serves

 How long the ingredients take to prepare

 How long the recipe takes to cook

top tips from our friends

We asked lots of Ella's Kitchen Friends for their best weaning advice. Here are their top four nuggets of wisdom:

 Go at your own pace: It's so easy to compare your baby to all the others you know, but every baby is different and will be ready for new experiences at different times. Let your little one set the pace.

 Love the mess: Messy little faces and sticky little hands are inevitable – and they are the best signs of a fun mealtime.

 The more the merrier: Parents, grandparents and siblings – let everyone take a turn helping during this exciting time in your baby's life; your baby will love it!

 Be kind to your time: Plan your meals, shop online or locally and learn recipe cheats (look out for our shortcuts) – that way you'll have extra time to really enjoy the weaning experience with your baby.

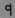

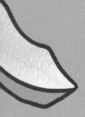

what is weaning?

Weaning is the really exciting time when little ones start to eat solid foods alongside their usual milk. It's sometimes called 'complementary feeding' because milk is still a really important source of nutrition but, over time, food is increasingly important to give little ones the nutrients they need to grow and develop. At the beginning, though, it's just about introducing a wide variety of tastes with milk providing most of the nutrients a little one needs.

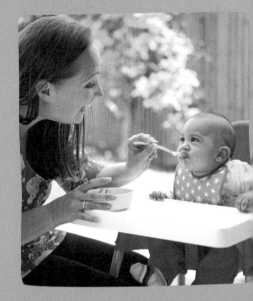

Introducing solids isn't just about making sure little ones have enough nutrition; solid foods, including finger foods, are essential for helping little ones learn to move foods around their mouths, to chew and pick up different-shaped foods. Weaning helps with motor skills development, too!

when to begin + signs your baby is ready

The UK's Department of Health and Social Care advises that most little ones are ready to start their foodie journey at 6 months. Until then, their usual milk provides all the nutrition they need.

Look out for the signs that your little one is ready for solid food. They should be able to:

☺ Stay in a sitting position and hold their head steady.

☺ Coordinate their hands, eyes and mouth so they can look at food, pick it up and pop it in their mouth.

☺ Swallow food rather than pushing it out with their tongue. (If they do this the first time you introduce solids, wait a few days and try again.)

If your baby chews their fists, wakes up more in the night than usual or wants extra milk feeds, that's just a sign that they're doing their baby thing! It's not a sign that they need to be weaned early.

If you think your little one is ready for solids earlier than 6 months of age, have a chat with your health visitor.

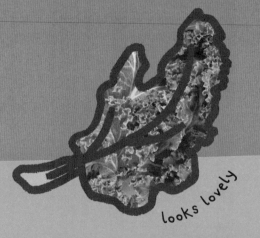

looks lovely

baby-led weaning or purees?

Baby-led weaning is an approach where little ones are given only finger foods and no purees or mashed texture foods from the very start of weaning. It's a great way to encourage hand-eye coordination and puts little ones in control of when they've had enough. However, it doesn't suit all little ones and it can be hard at first to ensure they're getting enough nutrients, especially iron.

For that reason, we recommend a mix-and-match approach where you offer pureed and mashed texture foods alongside finger foods so you can provide a wide range of nutrients, safe textures and finger foods to encourage motor skills development. But your weaning approach is a very personal thing and a decision to be taken with your little one in mind. It's totally up to you!

Take a look at our pull-out Weaning Meal Planner + Wall Chart for little ones aged 12 months+ in the middle of the book. It's perfect for decorating the fridge and keeping lots of essential weaning info to hand!

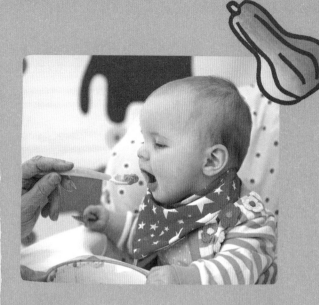

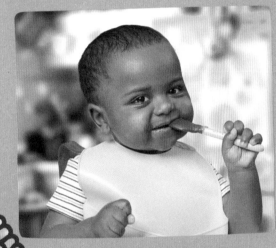

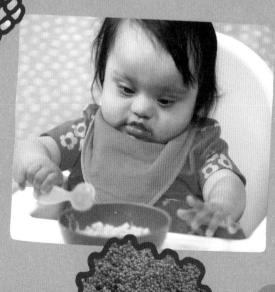

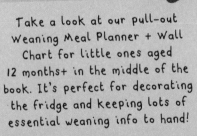

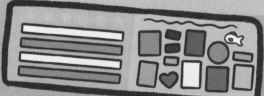

ages + stages

Little ones grow + develop suuuper fast in their first year. Here's some info on how babies learn to hold + eat a range of foods, so you'll know what foods to give + when to move on.

6 months

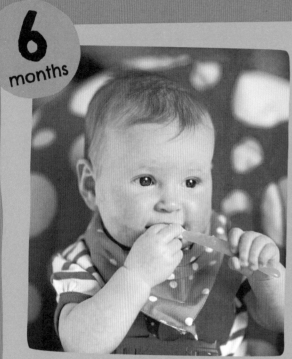

what can my baby do?

☺ Sit and hold head steady

☺ Pick up an object and bring it to their mouth

☺ Swallow food

☺ Hold stick-like finger food

what foods should I give?

☺ Smooth purees: start with a thin puree and gradually thicken it as your baby gets used to taking food from a spoon

☺ Finger foods the size and shape of an adult index finger which are soft enough to squish between thumb and finger, like a well-cooked carrot baton

what can my baby do?

☺ Sit independently

☺ Mash food against the roof of the mouth

☺ Control thumbs for holding finger food

what foods should I give?

☺ Thick purees with small, soft lumps, such as fork-mashed banana

☺ The same finger foods as for 6 months (see above)

7 months

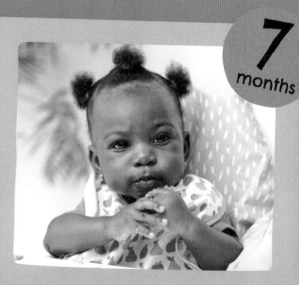

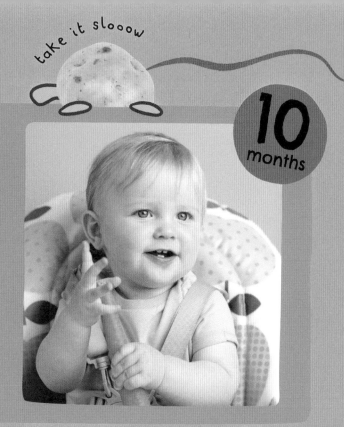

10 months

what can my baby do?

☺ Bite off and munch soft finger foods

☺ Pick up small, soft foods with pincer grip

what foods should I give?

☺ Thick purees with soft lumps the size of a pea

☺ Stick-like finger foods with soft, melty texture, such as cooked, peeled veggie sticks, well-cooked pasta pieces and well-cooked boiled egg slices

☺ Small, soft pincer-grip foods, such as chopped blueberries or raspberries

12 months

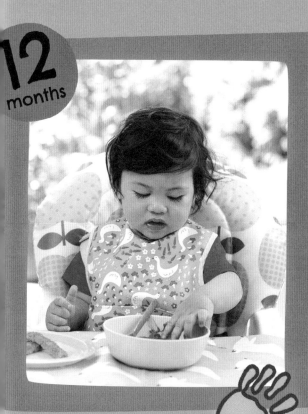

what can my baby do?

☺ Chew with a round and round motion to better cope with a wider range of textures

☺ Use simple cutlery

☺ Bite with more strength and accuracy

what foods should I give?

☺ Meals that are chopped up and served with minimal sauce/puree

☺ Cut round foods like grapes and cherry tomatoes into quarters

☺ Avoid foods with tough skins and gristle

☺ Avoid brittle, flaky, crumbly or hard foods

nutrition know-how

how to **balance** milk with food

For the first few months of weaning and beyond, milk is still a really important source of nutrients for little ones but, as they get older, food offers them more nutrients to fuel their super-fast growth and development.

When you start introducing solids for the first time, keep offering your baby's milk on demand and focus more on getting your little one used to eating without worrying about how much goes in. If they have a taste but most of it ends up in their hair and yours, that's fine!

Slowly build up how much you offer at one meal and then think about introducing a second meal after two or three weeks. Remember you don't need to rush; be led by your baby's pace. By the time your little one is 7–8 months old, you can offer three meals a day but snacks aren't needed until they're 12 months old. As your baby gets more of an appetite for foodie adventures, you'll find they naturally want less milk and you can think about dropping one or maybe two milk feeds but again, be led by your baby and make sure you offer a wide variety of yummy and nutritious foods.

Once your baby is confidently gobbling up their meals, be sure to still offer at least 600 ml/ 20 fl oz of their usual milk a day up to the age of 10 months. From 10–12 months, make sure your little one still gets 400 ml/14 fl oz of their usual milk a day. Little ones from 12 months old will be tucking into three meals and two nutritious snacks a day. You can either continue to breastfeed or offer 350 ml/12 fl oz of full-fat or semi-skimmed cows' milk or a fortified, no-added-sugar milk alternative alongside food.

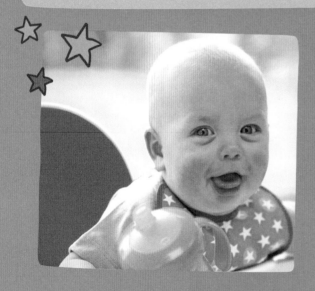

what **drinks** should I give my baby?

Babies only need their usual milk as a main drink when weaning with sips of water from a cup with meals, and throughout the day if it's hot. Juice or other drinks may contain lots of sugar, which can fill your baby up so they aren't hungry at mealtimes. Sugary drinks are also not kind to little teeth. Stick with milk and water and, if you do want to offer juice, make sure it's diluted well with water: one part juice to ten parts water is the recommendation.

key nutrients for weaning babies

It's important to offer a range of deeelicious foods with lots of variety so your little one gets a balanced diet. Variety is also super important for exciting tiny taste buds and can help little ones become more willing to try new foods when they're older. Here are some of the key nutrients to offer once your baby is eating a range of foods:

☺ **Protein** Found in meat, fish, eggs, pulses and soy products, protein is perfect for growing muscles and bones.

☺ **Carbohydrates** Foods rich in carbohydrate like oats, bread, pasta, couscous and other grains provide energy, fibre and some B vitamins to help your baby release energy from food.

☺ **Essential fats** These fats not only provide energy but also help little brains and eyes to develop. Essential fats can be found in foods like oily fish (salmon, mackerel and sardines), nuts and seeds (use finely ground nuts and seeds or nut butters) and avocado.

☺ **Iron** Your baby is born with a store of iron that lasts until around the age of 6 months. It's therefore important to provide iron in the weaning diet to help little brains and immune systems to develop. Iron can be found in red meat, lentils and other pulses, dried fruit like raisins and apricots, and green veg. Offer plant-based sources of iron with vitamin C from fruit or veg to help your baby absorb them.

☺ **Vitamin D** This isn't found in many foods and is formed in the skin when little ones are in the sunshine. It's important for bone growth and the immune system. The UK's Department of Health and Social Care recommends little ones under the age of 12 months who do not have 500 ml/18 fl oz or more of infant formula a day take a vitamin D supplement, providing 8.5–10 micrograms of vitamin D (along with vitamins A and C). You can buy drops especially made for babies and there are free supplements available if you are on a low income. Once babies are a year old, they should have a supplement offering 10 micrograms of vitamin D.

tweet beet

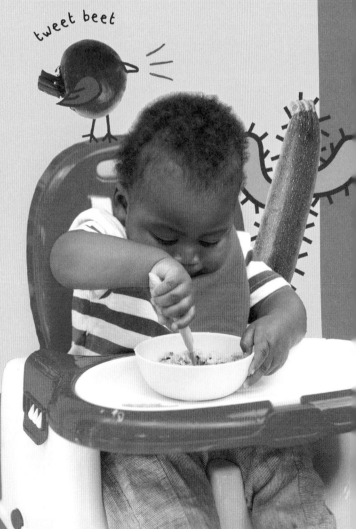

To ensure your baby is getting all their essential nutrients, pick foods from each of the food groups.

growing a little veggie or vegan

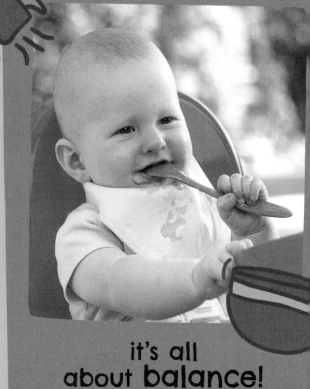

There is no reason why you can't provide a balanced, yummy, plant-based diet for your baby but make sure you pack in a range of protein sources throughout the day (lentils, beans, soy, nut butters or ground nuts, seeds and a variety of grains) so your little one has enough for growing up big and strong. Watch out for key vitamins and minerals too!

☺ **Calcium** Needed for growing bones and teeth, calcium is found in dairy foods but plant-based sources include nuts and seeds (ground or as butter), especially sesame and chia seeds, green veg like broccoli, spinach and kale, dried fruit like figs, bread, calcium-set tofu and fortified dairy alternatives.

☺ **Vitamin B12** This vitamin helps to keep the heart, blood cells and nervous system healthy and is found in foods of animal origin like milk, eggs and meat. If your little one is eating a plant-based diet, you might want to consider a vitamin B12 supplement but chat with your health visitor first.

☺ **Vitamin D** See page 15.

☺ **Iodine** This is an important mineral for growth and thyroid function but it is only found in white fish and milk, so again, consider a supplement for babies following a plant-based diet.

☺ **Iron** See page 15 for advice on plant-based iron sources.

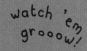

watch 'em grooow!

it's all about balance!

Once your little one is tucking into at least one meal a day, try to pack in all the important food groups: carbohydrates, protein and dairy foods (or alternatives), plus veggies and fruit. Every meal doesn't have to include every food group but try to provide balance and variety as much as you can throughout the day. Some ideas are:

☺ **Mashed minced beef with sweet potato + grated cheese, served with steamed broccoli** (protein + carbohydrate + dairy + 2 veg)

☺ **Mashed tuna pasta bake with tomato-based sauce + steamed carrot sticks** (protein + carbohydrate + 2 veg)

☺ **Porridge with a dollop of Greek yogurt + grated apple** (carbohydrate + dairy + fruit)

☺ **Pitta fingers with hummus, cucumber sticks + banana fingers** (carbohydrate + protein + veg + fruit)

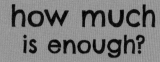

variety is the spice of life

A wide variety of foods simply means offering more than one or two types of each food group to make tiny taste buds tingle and provide a broader range of nutrients. The more variety you give your baby, the more likely they are to accept new foods when they're older. Try to offer some of these foods if you can:

Carbohydrates – bread (wholemeal, rye, pitta, etc.), pasta (white, brown, lentil), rice (white, brown or a mix), potatoes (standard, sweet potato), grains (oats, quinoa, buckwheat, etc.).

Proteins – meat, fish, eggs, lentils, beans (cannellini beans, chickpeas and products like hummus, butter beans, haricot beans, red kidney beans, etc.), soy products like tofu.

Dairy – milk, yogurt, cheese and fortified milk alternatives.

Fruit + veg – eating a rainbow of tasty veg and fruits isn't just nutritious, it's also super fun for the senses! Try red tomatoes, orange carrots, yellow melon, green broccoli, purple blueberries and white cauliflower. Stick a rainbow chart up in the kitchen and tick off the colours your little one has eaten all week.

Healthy fats – nut butters, seeds, oils like olive or rapeseed oil, avocado, oily fish like salmon and sardines (canned are just as nutritious as fresh).

how much is enough?

The portion sizes in this book are just a guide. Little ones' appetites will vary from one day to another, depending upon growth spurts, teething or being poorly, so don't worry if some days they don't eat much and others they never stop! It's what they eat over a week or two that's more important than each individual meal. As long as your baby is eating a variety of foods and growing well, you don't need to worry about whether they didn't eat much at breakfast one day.

Your baby is reeeally good at knowing when they've had enough to eat. If you're spoon-feeding, they'll turn their head away, spit the food out or push away the spoon. If they're eating finger foods, they'll stop eating, want to get out of the high chair or start throwing or dropping food. These signs let you know that they're full. If you've gently encouraged them two or three times and your little one has said no, it's time to end the meal.

In short, you decide what and when your baby eats and your little one decides whether to eat and how much. Trust your baby and your own instinct!

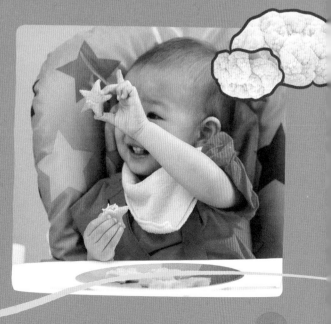

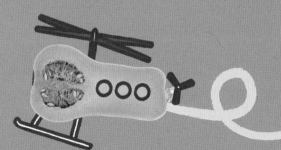

creating a healthy relationship with food

The eating habits your little one learns in the first year or two of life can often last into later childhood + beyond so get off to a flying start by offering super-yummy, healthy foods from the beginning!

the importance of veg in weaning

Studies have shown that offering a wide variety of single vegetables in the first few weeks and throughout weaning, either as purees or finger foods, can help little ones learn to accept veg, and that this habit can be carried through into later life. Offer a rainbow of veg, among other foods, and make sure you include some of the more savoury-tasting veg like broccoli, cauliflower and green beans, as well as sweeter ones like carrot or parsnip.

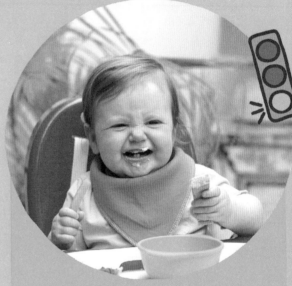

keep going!

The first time your little one tries a food, especially if it tastes a little bit bitter like broccoli, they might pull a funny face. It doesn't mean they don't like it or won't learn to accept it. It just means it's new and surprising. Keep the camera at the ready for those first taste faces and remember, it can take around ten tries of a new food before it's accepted so don't give up!

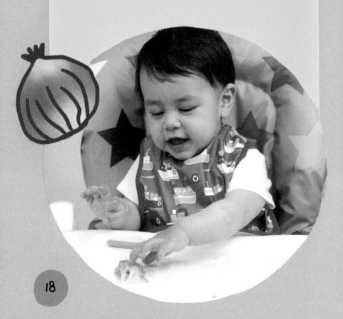

setting a routine

Little ones don't need a strict feeding timetable but having an eating routine where the flow of events is consistent on most days gives them a structure, which can be comforting. This could be as simple as the following:

☺ Waking up: Usual milk

☺ Mid-morning: Usual milk

☺ Lunchtime: Veggie puree or finger food

☺ Mid-afternoon: Usual milk

☺ Teatime: Usual milk

☺ Bedtime: Usual milk

This flow will change over time as you offer more meals and fewer milk feeds so settle on what works for you and try to keep it consistent most days, though things will obviously change on days out, weekends or holidays – and that's fine!

happy mealtimes

It can be easy to feel the pressure when life is busy, budgets are stretched and your little one is being fussy. But if you're stressed at mealtimes, your baby will pick up on it so try to stay calm, even if they reject the food you've just spent ages preparing. Remember, it's not a reflection on your cooking! If your baby rejects their meal, calmly take it away and try again a bit later. Don't offer a sweet treat or an alternative meal or your baby will quickly learn that they get pudding if they turn their nose up at dinner!

livin' on the veg

little copy cats

Little ones love to copy those around them, so try to eat healthily in front of them most of the time, if you can. In fact, eating together is a great way to demonstrate your own healthy habits. It tells your baby that mealtimes are about enjoyment, fun and social family time as well as eating. Of course, it's not always possible to eat together when little ones eat early and everyone is busy. But when your baby is eating, try to eat a small snack that's similar to their food so they can feel involved. For example, if they're having carrots with a meal, why not eat some carrot sticks at the same time?

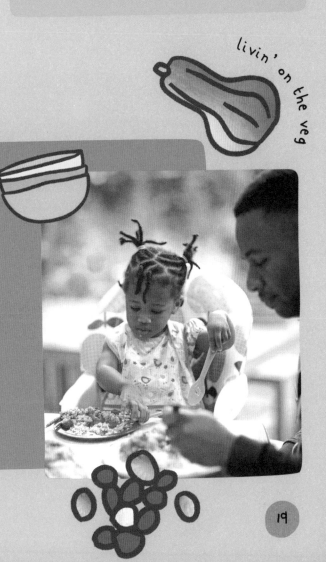

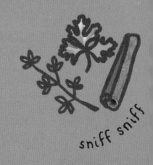

sniff sniff

tasty, squishy food play

Sensory food play is a reeeally fun way for little ones to familiarize themselves with food outside of mealtimes. Research shows that engaging with food using all the senses (sight, touch, smell, taste and sound), without any pressure to eat, helps little ones learn about the different shapes, colours, sizes, textures and even sounds of food, which can make them more curious to try new foods at mealtimes.

The early years are a time of super-speedy development for little ones and the habits gained in the first two years of life can be carried into later childhood and beyond. If little ones learn to like healthy foods like vegetables early in life, they are more likely to continue eating them as they grow up. One of the ways to help little ones learn to accept vegetables is through repeatedly eating or experiencing them. It can take ten tries of a new food, particularly vegetables, before it is accepted, which sounds a lot, but even touching the food, having it on the plate or tasting it with their tongue still counts so get those senses tingling!

You'll find lots of fun sensory activities throughout the book to try with your little one when you're making the yummy recipes, so keep an eye out!

mythbusting

is sensory food play wasteful?

You don't need to waste any food that's used in sensory play. Just by seeing, holding, smelling or even hearing foods as they're prepared and cooked is enough to stimulate the senses to then encourage little ones to have a taste at mealtimes.

is it time consuming?

While it's fantastic if you have the time to plan more elaborate sensory activities, it can be as simple as holding up a banana to your face like a smile, giving your baby a pointy, bumpy carrot to feel or sitting them with you in the kitchen while you cook, listening to the sizzle of frying onions and smelling the yummy foodie aromas.

is it messy?

Making a mess is a great way for little ones to learn about their foodie world but some little ones aren't keen on getting messy or touching foods that are slimy or squishy. And you might not always fancy clearing up afterwards. Exploring whole veg and fruit with all the senses before you prepare them is a mess-free way to avoid waste yet still get the benefits of sensory exploration.

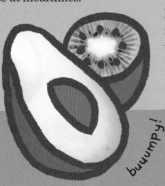

buuumpy!

good in every sense

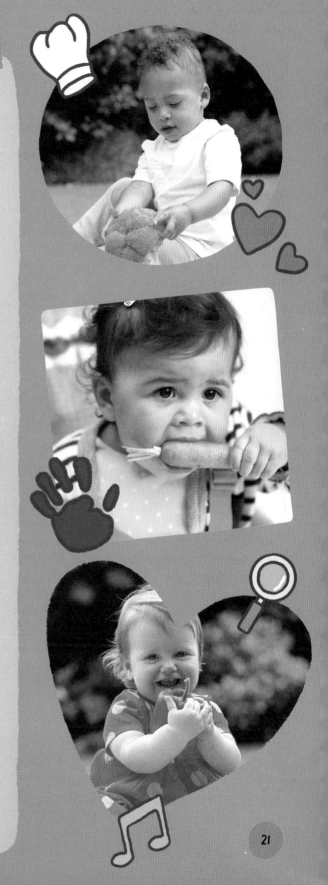

tastes terrific

Some fruits and veggies taste a little more sweet, sour or bitter than others. Little ones may react with strong and even funny faces at first but that's because everything is new. Keep trying with those new tastes to help your baby learn to accept them. Adding herbs and spices to food is a great way to get little taste buds tingling.

smells super

You baby's sense of smell and taste are closely linked and delicious foodie aromas can trigger hunger so it's really important to get those little noses twitching in fun and enjoyable ways.

feels fantastic

Letting your baby explore whole fruit and veg with their hands can help to familiarize them with the touchy-feely textures of new foods, from furry kiwi to bobbly broccoli. Learning about food through touch outside of mealtimes can help stimulate little ones' curiosity to try those foods when it comes to eating.

looks lovely

If food looks interesting, colourful and fun, little ones might be more keen to try it. Offer a rainbow of fruits and veggies across the week and show your baby how they look before you prepare them for eating so they can see the different shapes, sizes, colours and textures.

sounds sensational

Foodie sounds can create excitement for a meal, from the bubble of soup or the sizzle of onions to the deeelicious crunch of the first bite of toast. Our sense of hearing really adds to the eating experience so let your little one sit in the kitchen with you while you're cooking so they can experience the sounds, smells and sights before mealtime!

allergies + safety

introducing allergens during weaning

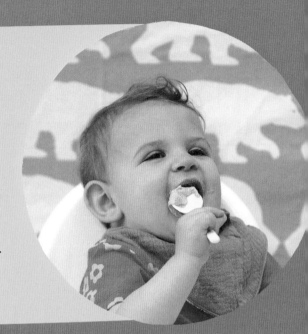

Some foods can cause an allergic response in a small number of babies. Allergies to foods are more common in families with a history of food and other allergies, like hay fever or eczema, but they are still quite rare.

An allergic reaction can be immediate or delayed. We've included lots of information on page 24 on how to spot and deal with an allergic response in your little one.

what are allergens?

The most common allergen foods are:

☺ cereals containing gluten

☺ eggs

☺ fish

☺ crustaceans like prawns and crab

☺ molluscs like mussels and oysters

☺ nuts

☺ peanuts

☺ soy + soy products

☺ celery + celeriac

☺ cows' milk + dairy products

☺ mustard

☺ sesame seeds

☺ sulphur dioxide (a preservative in some drinks + foods like dried fruit)

☺ lupin (a legume, like peanut)

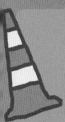

when + how to introduce allergen foods

Introduce allergen foods in small but regular amounts, from around the age of 6 months. Offer them one at a time, when your baby is feeling well and in teeny tiny amounts (a quarter to a half of a teaspoon) so you can spot any allergic reactions.

Try to introduce a new allergen early in the day so you can watch out for any reactions for a few hours afterwards. Breakfast or mid-morning is a good idea. For example, if you start with cows' milk, add a small amount of milk or plain yogurt (just a quarter to a half of a teaspoon) to a veggie or fruit puree you've given your baby before and mix well before giving to your little one.

tips on prep of allergen foods

Follow the tips below for offering allergen foods with a safe texture for little ones:

☺ **Nuts + seeds** – finely ground or as a butter and added to purees and cereals/porridge

☺ **Fish, shellfish + molluscs** – well-cooked; check carefully for bones; puree, chop, flake or mash

☺ **Wheat + cereals containing gluten** – oats as porridge (can be blended), couscous, toast or bread fingers, pasta pieces

bee safe!

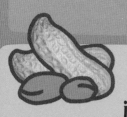

new research on introducing egg + peanut

New studies have shown that introducing egg and peanut early, from 4 months (if they are ready and under the advice of a health professional), can reduce the risk of developing an allergy to those foods in those babies with a family history of allergies. However, you must always speak with an allergy specialist before introducing any allergen foods before the age of 6 months and if your little one is at risk of food allergies.

For babies who are not at risk of food allergies, the advice on egg and peanut is to introduce small amounts of well-cooked, hard-boiled, pureed egg, added to a familiar food, from 6 months of age. Once you are sure that egg

is tolerated by your baby, you can think about introducing peanut.

Whole nuts shouldn't be given to children under the age of 5 years because they're a choking risk. Peanut butter on its own is quite sticky so can also be a choking risk, so, for a first experience of peanut, try smooth peanut butter (no added sugar or salt) or ground peanuts mixed with a familiar puree.

If peanut and egg are tolerated without any reactions, aim to offer each food regularly, as with other allergen foods.

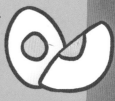

remember, reactions can be immediate or delayed

Keep an eye out for any reactions – check out the list below for some of the signs of an allergic reaction and what to do if your baby has one. If your baby has no reactions, you can start to build up the amount of that allergen gradually. Offer it regularly – at least once or twice a week.

Wait 2–3 days before introducing another allergen food like egg, soy or nuts. Chat to your health visitor or doctor about introducing allergens if you have a family history of allergies.

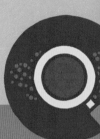

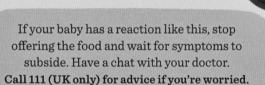

baby food allergies

signs of an immediate reaction

An immediate reaction, which usually occurs within 30 minutes of eating the food, may be mild, like:

☹ Irritated or itchy skin rash (such as hives), especially around your baby's face

☹ Swollen lips, face or eyes

☹ Tummy pain, diarrhoea or vomiting

☹ Worsening of eczema or asthma symptoms

If your baby has a reaction like this, don't offer the allergen food again and dial a medical helpline such as 111 (UK only) for advice, or speak with your doctor.

If your baby has a swollen tongue, persistent cough, difficulty breathing or is pale, floppy or unconscious, **dial an emergency medical helpline such as 999 (UK only) right away for help.**

signs of a delayed reaction

It's important to note that not all allergic reactions are immediate and your little one may have a delayed food reaction, which may not cause symptoms for several hours after the food has been eaten.

Symptoms of a delayed reaction, usually seen 2–72 hours after consuming the trigger food:

☹ Recurring tummy pains, bloating, vomiting or reflux

☹ Diarrhoea

☹ Colic or wind

☹ Worsening eczema (if present)

If your baby has a reaction like this, stop offering the food and wait for symptoms to subside. Have a chat with your doctor. **Call 111 (UK only) for advice if you're worried.**

If you are concerned at all about allergies or offering allergens, have a chat with your health visitor or doctor first.

tips on texture + choking

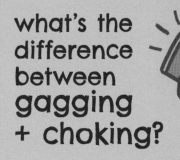

Each recipe has been carefully created to offer just the right texture to help little ones develop chewing skills and hand-eye coordination while being safe and avoiding any choking risks. Check out the advice at the beginning of each chapter, which goes into lots more detail on getting food texture, shape and size just right for little ones at each stage of their development.

More generally, it's important to avoid giving babies the following foods:

☺ **Round foods:** Grapes, cherry tomatoes and sausages need to be chopped into quarters, lengthways, as they can be a choking risk. Only give these to older babies, from 12 months +, even if chopped.

☺ **Hard foods:** Nuts, popcorn or foods with hard or shiny skin like peas, sweetcorn and peppers can be a choking risk, as can hard raw fruit and veg like carrots or apples. Chop up foods with hard skins, such as peppers, into small pieces. Cook them well, along with foods like peas and sweetcorn, and offer them as part of a mixed meal that has a thick sauce or puree, such as a stew or potato-topped pie, from 10–12 months +. Hard raw fruit and veg like carrots or apples shouldn't be given to babies unless they are finely grated and even then, best from 10 months onwards. Whole nuts should be avoided before the age of 5 years.

☺ **Flaky, brittle or crumbly foods:** Foods that break up easily into small, hard pieces like flapjacks, crisps or hard biscuits can be a choking risk. It's best to go for finger foods that melt easily in the mouth and can be squished between your thumb and finger, without falling apart into hard chunks.

what's the difference between gagging + choking?

Gagging: It's perfectly normal for babies to gag as soft, little pieces of food move to the back of their tongues. It can be quite scary to watch but a baby's gagging reflex is far more sensitive than an adult's. You may see them go red and start coughing or spluttering and their tongue may thrust forward. Through gagging, your baby's clever body moves the food forward for another go at chewing and swallowing or for spitting out. Try not to worry – keep smiling and reassure your baby that everything is OK.

Choking: This happens when a piece of food has slipped down and got stuck in your baby's windpipe. They may go quiet and even start to go blue. If this happens and your little one is not coughing to bring the food back up, start the baby choking sequence to dislodge the object (talk to your health visitor or do a baby first-aid course for what to do in this scenario). To prevent choking, never leave your baby alone while eating and never offer any food that could be a choking risk (see left for examples).

beep beep!

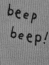

foods to avoid

⊗ Added salt: Little ones under a year old need less than 1 g of salt – or 0.4 g of sodium – a day, so added salt is a no-no. Look out! Processed foods not intended for babies, such as pasta sauces and breakfast cereals, could have lots of added salt in them; and stock cubes, too.

⊗ Added sugar: Your baby is sweet enough, so avoid adding sugar in your cooking. Natural sugars in fruits provide plenty of sweetness – any more could lead to tooth decay or an unhealthy sweet tooth.

⊗ Honey: Bears may like honey, but little ones shouldn't try it until they reach a year old, as it contains bacteria that could be harmful to tiny tummies.

⊗ Whole nuts: Whole nuts, including peanuts, are easy to choke on. Don't give them until your child is over 5 years old.

⊗ Low-fat foods: Low-fat yogurt, fromage frais, cheese and spreads aren't ideal for little ones. Babies have tiny tummies but are growing fast, so need energy-dense foods like full-fat yogurt and cheese to fuel their rapid growth. You may be able to introduce low-fat foods once your child is 2 years old, as long as they are growing well.

⊗ Some fish + shellfish: Some fish, including shark, marlin and swordfish, can contain high levels of mercury. Avoid giving these for the first year and after that only in small amounts. Shellfish can carry a risk of food poisoning if it's undercooked, so be very, very careful to cook it properly all the way through!

⊗ Eggs: It's now OK to give a runny egg, for example with soldiers, if your baby is okay with eating eggs and if the egg has a lion stamp (UK only). If it doesn't, then make sure it's well cooked before giving it to babies.

⊗ Unpasteurized + blue cheeses: Soft, unpasteurized cheeses, such as Brie and Camembert, and 'mouldy' or 'blue' cheeses, such as Stilton, carry a small risk of food poisoning and are best saved for after your baby's all-important first birthday. It's OK to give unpasteurized cheeses if they're cooked into a meal though.

⊗ Rice drinks: These aren't suitable as a substitute for breastmilk or formula milk or for cows' milk over 12 months because they can contain too much of a heavy metal called arsenic. Rice and rice products are OK, as the levels of arsenic are tightly controlled, but it's best to avoid rice drinks if your little one is under 5 years old.

frrreezing

Batch cooking and freezing is a great time saver. You can freeze purees and mashed meals in ice cube trays or little weaning bowls with lids. Just follow these tips for safe freezing:

☺ Make sure your purees are completely cooled before you put them in the freezer (see opposite).

☺ Label the containers with the recipe and date you made it.

☺ Use frozen food within a month.

☺ Defrost food completely before reheating it. The safest way to do this is in the fridge overnight or in the microwave.

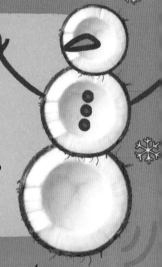

brrrr!

safe + secure

Following a few simple rules helps keep little ones as safe as possible on their weaning adventure.

Wipe clean: Keep surfaces, chopping boards and utensils spotlessly clean. Use separate chopping boards for meat and veg.

Clean hands: Always wash your own hands before preparing any food. Then check that your baby's hands are clean before eating. It's never too early to get into the habit of hand-washing before a meal.

Wash, peel + scrape: Wash all your ingredients and either peel or scrub away tough skins before you cook.

Clean bowls + spoons: If your baby is younger than 6 months, sterilize all your feeding equipment (see page 28). After that, just make sure everything is washed really well in hot, soapy water and rinsed in clean water.

Hot, hot, hot: Cook or reheat food so that it's piping hot all the way through, then stir it and cool it to a lukewarm temperature. Test it against your bottom lip to make sure it's just right for your baby. Never reheat cooked food more than once, and never refreeze food that's been frozen and then defrosted.

Two's company: Never leave your baby alone when eating or drinking – you need to be around in case of any mishaps, including choking (see page 25).

Be cool: If you want to refrigerate (or freeze) food, make sure it's completely cold first. Cool it quickly – within 2 hours of cooking – by standing the container of food in a bowl of cold water. Once it's completely cold, pop it in the fridge (or freezer – see tips opposite).

Store safely: Keep cooked and raw meats covered and away from each other. Place cooked foods above raw foods in the fridge, and put non-meat foods on a separate fridge shelf.

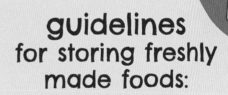

guidelines
for storing freshly made foods:

☺ **In the fridge:** 2 days in an airtight container

☺ **In the freezer:** Store at -18°C/0°F. Try to use frozen food within a month

☺ **Cakes + bakes:** In the cupboard for up to 3–4 days in an airtight container

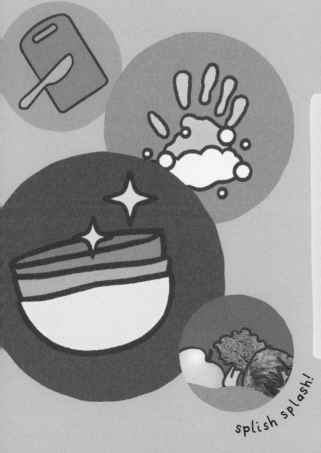

splish splash!

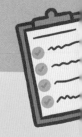

practical tips

your weaning kitchen

So, before you get started, here's our guide to a few essentials you'll need in your kitchen to make it easier to prepare and store your baby's food.

☺ **Vegetable peeler** because you'll be doing a lot of peeling

☺ **Sharp paring knife** to chop things up nice and small or for cutting up finger foods

☺ **Small saucepans** that are perfect sizes for reheating little portions

☺ **Steamer**...but that needs a section all of its own (see opposite)

☺ **Sieve** to strain fruit, catch naughty pips and help get rid of tough skins

☺ **Hand blender** or food processor if you're making purees, to whiz your baby's food to the right texture (food processors are better for tougher skins on veggies)

☺ **Potato masher** for when your little one moves on from puree

☺ **Sterilizer** for spoons and bowls, but only if you're weaning before your baby is 6 months old (you can sterilize in boiling water if you would prefer)

☺ **Ice cube trays** for storing purees in the freezer in portions

☺ **Freezer bags** for storing frozen puree cubes, or for freezing finger foods

☺ **Labels + marker pen** so that you know what's what and when you made it

☺ **Beakers + cups** to help your baby move on from a bottle

☺ **Spoons + bowls** for feeding time itself

☺ **High chair** or booster seat so that your little one can sit at the table

☺ **Bibs** – we like the wipeable ones with a pocket to catch the bits

☺ **Face cloths or muslins** for wiping messy hands and faces

menu planning

Making a weekly plan of what you're going to eat as a family can help save time and money. Once your little one is on their weaning journey, eating one, two or more meals a day, you can apply the same principles to their diet as you do with your own to help ensure you're all getting variety and balance. See our pull-out weaning meal planner + wall chart for little ones aged 12 months+ in the middle of the book for more details. Once your baby is 12 months old, try to offer the following each day:

☺ 5 portions of carbohydrate foods

☺ 5 portions of fruit or veg

☺ 3 portions of dairy foods

☺ 2 portions of protein foods (3 if vegetarian or vegan)

See page 16 for ideas on how to offer a variety of each food type.

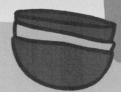

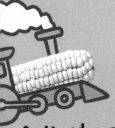

full steam ahead!

Steaming food is the best way to preserve nutrients and keep taste locked in. For making purees or first finger foods, steam veg until they're soft enough to squish between your thumb and finger. Veg should be cut into the size and shape of your index finger if you're giving them straight to your little one.

types of steamers

Dedicated steamer: Some steamers are fancy electrical tiered units, while others look like a stack of saucepans with holes in.

Steamer basket: These are holey baskets with little feet – they look like tiny spaceships! You put them in a saucepan with a little boiling water, cover and steam away.

Colander: Pop your colander in a pan with a little water and cover it with a lid.

Microwave: Put a little water in a microwave-safe bowl, add the veggies and cover with clingfilm. Pierce the film and then zap in the microwave until the veggies are tender (about 2–3 minutes for leafy greens and 5–6 minutes for chopped root veg – but check your user guide).

steam roasting

You can also use a clever mode of cooking called steam roasting. It works really well with all sorts of veggies and even meat or fish like chicken and salmon. You simply roast the food in a tin like you would normally but you cover the dish or tray with foil until the last 10 minutes of cooking. This keeps the moisture in so the food has a deeelicious roasted taste but without the crispy, dry bits that might be a choking risk.

it's not a race!

Don't worry if your friend's baby is munching mash or tackling finger foods before yours. All little ones are different and will progress at their own pace. Milestone charts are just a guide and it's important to focus on your own baby and not worry too much about comparing them with others. Trust your instincts. If you are concerned with your baby's progress, then have a chat with your health visitor but avoid comparisons with others!

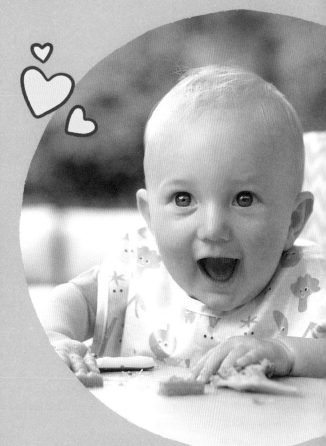

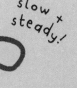

slow + steady!

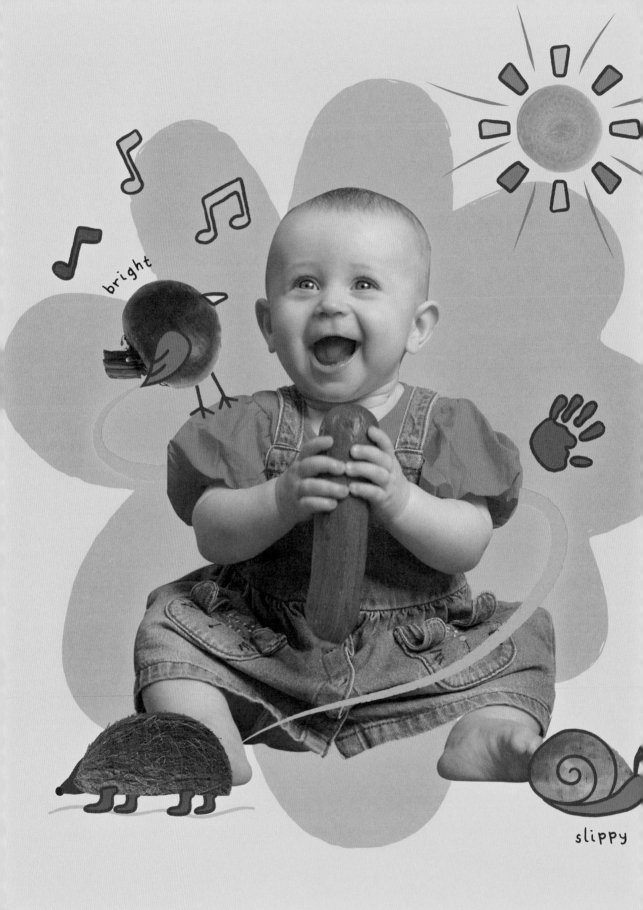

bright

slippy

from
6
months

tangy!

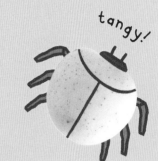

ready, steady, weeean!

bobbly

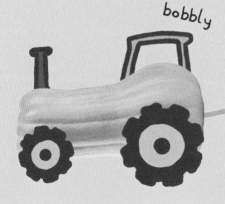

the first week

Once you've identified the signs that your little one is ready to wean (see page 10), you're ready to get started. Here's all the essential information you need to make sure you both put your best weaning feet forward.

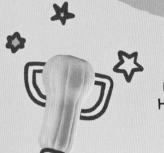

best first foods

Research shows that offering babies a variety of single veg, repeatedly and in variety, early on and throughout weaning is a great way to help them learn to accept and even like vegetables, not just now but potentially in years to come, too. Our planner on page 34 shows you how to try this 'veg-led' weaning approach.

Babies are used to the taste of breastmilk or their usual formula milk, which is quite sweet, so savoury tastes might be a bit of a surprise at first. Your baby might pull all sorts of funny and even disgusted faces on the first taste of a new food but go gently and keep offering that food. It can take about ten tries before it's accepted.

time for liftoff!

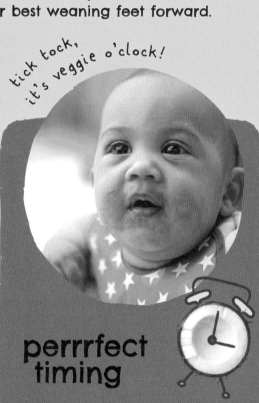

tick tock, it's veggie o'clock!

perrrfect timing

Offer your baby their first foods at a time when they're well and not too tired or hungry. Relax, leave plenty of time and don't start weaning if you've planned a busy day. Just after a post-nap milk feed is a great time.

Offer a small amount of puree on a spoon or a single stick of cooked veg. If your baby pushes the food back out with their tongue, wait a day or two and try again.

how much?

At first, it's all about offering a variety of tiny tastes to tempt tiny taste buds so your little one might only eat a spoonful or two of puree or one or two cooked veggie sticks. Continue to give your baby's usual milk on demand as this provides all their nutrition for now. They'll build up the amount of food they eat over time. If you've frozen puree in ice cube trays then you will probably only need to defrost one cube at a time for the first few days. Check out page 26 for how to defrost safely.

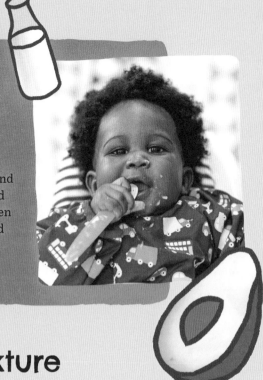

nice 'n' runny

tips on texture

At 6 months of age, your baby can move their tongue up and down to move food to the back of their mouth for swallowing. They will independently open their mouth when a spoon is offered. They can also hold a finger-like object, such as a carrot stick, in their palm so it peeps out of their fist for eating. With this in mind, follow our handy texture tips.

Purees: Start by offering a relatively thin puree, the texture of runny honey and super-smooth without lumps. It should fall off a spoon in dollops. You'll probably need to loosen the texture of any purees you make with either your baby's usual milk or cooking water. In some cases, you'll need to pass the puree through a sieve to remove fibrous bits. We've lots of recipes and tips on pages 34–53. After a couple of weeks, you can thicken the texture by adding less liquid.

Finger foods: These are a great way to encourage hand-eye coordination from 6 months of age. Chop veggies and fruits into sticks the size and shape of your index finger and steam until they're soft enough to squish easily between your thumb and forefinger. Soft fruits like banana won't need cooking. Make sure that any finger foods you offer are super-melty and don't crumble, flake or break into small pieces that might be a choking risk.

steam me!

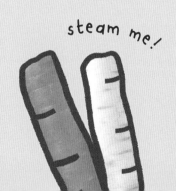

smoooothly does it!

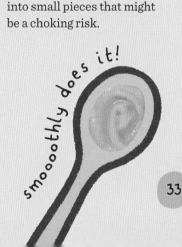

our first tastes
weaning planner

We know those very first steps on your baby's weaning journey can feel a bit daunting and even scary. To help you, we've created a handy planner for the first week, using the veg-led weaning approach (see page 18). Keep mealtimes positive, be led by their appetite and have lots of foodie fun to help build your baby's relationship with food.

	day 1	day 2	day 3	day 4	day 5	day 6	day 7
week 1	broccoli	cauliflower	carrots	green beans	broccoli	cauliflower	carrots

Start with 1–2 spoonfuls or 1–2 batons just after lunchtime milk (or whatever time suits you and your baby best!), building up day by day, led by your baby's appetite. Finger foods should be the size and shape of your index finger and cooked so that they're soft enough to squish easily. Green beans are stringy so best served pureed. Avoid giving hard foods like raw apple or carrot or food with tough and shiny skins as finger foods.

using the planner

We suggest mixing up the veg you offer your little one each day but also offering the same veg repeatedly so your baby can get familiar with it. Remember, it can take up to ten tries of a new food before it's accepted, so keep going! The recipes for these purees and more can be found on pages 36–39 but there's handy advice on page 40 for how to cut and cook finger foods if you'd rather offer those.

after the first week

Keep offering single veg as purees or finger foods until your little one accepts them. When you feel ready, you can move on to combinations of veg in purees and offer fruit (as puree or finger food), along with other foods, as explained in the next chapter.

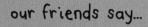

our friends say...

'I wanted my baby to associate her high chair with having lots of fun so in the week before we started weaning, I'd sit her in it to play games and sing songs. Then, when the food came, she knew that was going to be fun, too!'

be a veggie explorer!

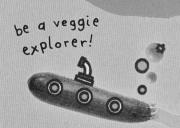

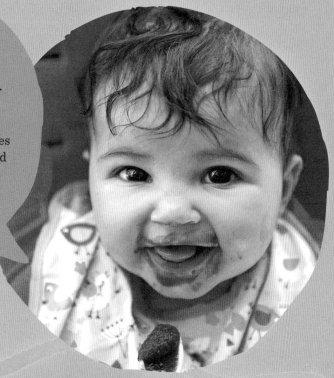

other exciting veg to try

Eating a rainbow of veg is a fantastic way to excite tiny taste buds. Below are some other yummy veggie tastes to try and you'll find the recipes on pages 36–39. You can also offer fruits as long as they're peeled and steamed until squishable and then pureed with your baby's usual milk or offered as finger foods. Banana can just be mashed with a little of their usual milk until smooth or cut into fingers for little hands to hold. Soft fruits like strawberries or kiwi don't need to be steamed. Just remove any stems, peel or pithy bits and cut into fingers.

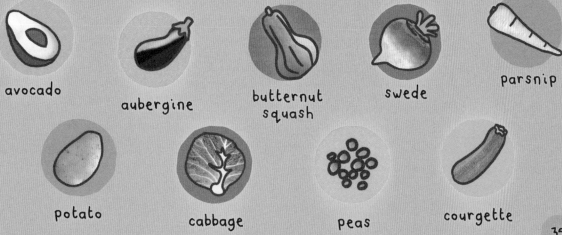

avocado

aubergine

butternut squash

swede

parsnip

potato

cabbage

peas

courgette

35

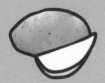

potato

makes **20** spoons

cook **20** mins

1 **potato** (about 200 g/7 oz), such as Maris Piper, peeled and cut into 1 cm/1/2 inch cubes

60 ml/21/2 fl oz **baby's usual milk**

Cook the potato in a small saucepan of boiling water for 20 minutes or until very tender, then drain. Transfer the potato to a bowl and gradually add the milk, mashing with a fork between each addition until the puree is loose enough that a little on the end of a spoon falls off sideways without any shaking.

broccoli

makes **20** spoons

cook **10** mins

1/2 small head **broccoli** (about 125 g/ 41/2 oz), cut into small florets

2–3 tablespoons **baby's usual milk**

Steam or boil the broccoli in a saucepan over a medium heat for 8 minutes or until very tender. Adding the milk, puree the broccoli in a food processor, or using a hand blender, until smooth.

cauliflower

makes **30** spoons

cook **10** mins

1/3 small head **cauliflower** (about 140 g/ 5 oz), cut into small florets

4–5 tablespoons **baby's usual milk**

Steam or boil the cauliflower in a saucepan over a medium heat for 8–10 minutes until very tender. Adding the milk, puree the cauliflower in a food processor, or using a hand blender, until smooth.

green beans

makes **20** spoons

cook **20** mins

100 g/31/2 oz **green beans**, trimmed and halved

3–4 tablespoons **baby's usual milk**

Steam or boil the beans in a saucepan over a medium heat for 7 minutes or until very tender. Gradually adding the milk, puree the beans in a food processor, or using a hand blender, until smooth. Pass the puree through a sieve to remove any fibrous pieces before serving.

cabbage

makes **15** spoons

cook **5** mins

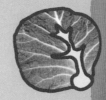

1/4 **white cabbage** (about 125 g/4 1/2 oz), cored and finely chopped

2–3 tablespoons **baby's usual milk**

Steam or boil the cabbage in a saucepan over a medium heat for 5 minutes or until very tender. Adding the milk, puree the cabbage in a food processor, or using a hand blender, until smooth. Pass the puree through a sieve to remove any fibrous pieces before serving.

avocado

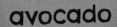

serves **1**

cook **no cook**

1 very ripe **avocado**, peeled, stoned and chopped

Baby's usual milk (optional)

Using the back of a fork, mash the avocado until completely smooth, adding a little of your baby's usual milk if necessary. Alternatively, puree using a hand blender. (Mashed avocado won't keep, so discard any leftovers.)

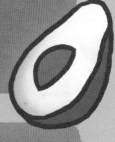

peas

makes **30** spoons

cook **15** mins

150 g/5 1/2 oz **frozen peas**

3–4 tablespoons **baby's usual milk**

Steam or boil the peas in a saucepan over a medium heat for 10–12 minutes until completely tender. Puree the peas with the milk in a food processor, or using a hand blender, until completely smooth. Pass the puree through a sieve to remove any pieces of skin, if necessary.

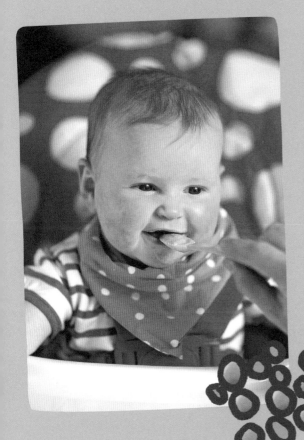

37

courgette

makes **20** spoons
cook **10** mins

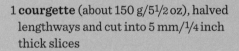

1 **courgette** (about 150 g/5½ oz), halved lengthways and cut into 5 mm/¼ inch thick slices

Steam or boil the courgette in a saucepan over a medium heat for 8–10 minutes until completely tender. Puree in a food processor, or using a hand blender, until it is smooth.

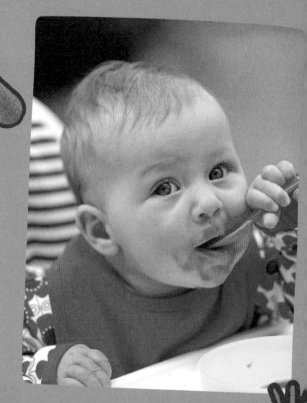

aubergine

makes **35** spoons
cook **10** mins

1 **aubergine** (about 250 g/9 oz), cut into 1 cm/½ inch cubes

2–3 tablespoons **baby's usual milk**

Steam the aubergine in a saucepan over a medium heat for 10 minutes or until the skin and flesh are completely tender. Puree the aubergine with the milk in a food processor, or using a hand blender, until smooth. Pass the puree through a sieve to remove any pieces of skin, if necessary.

carrots

makes **30** spoons
cook **15** mins

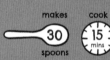

3 **carrots** (about 250 g/9 oz), peeled and halved lengthways

3–4 tablespoons **baby's usual milk**

Slice the carrots into half-moon shapes, 5 mm/¼ inch thick. Steam or boil the carrots in a saucepan over a medium heat for 10–12 minutes until completely tender. Puree the carrots with the milk in a food processor, or using a hand blender, until completely smooth.

parsnips

makes **30** spoons cook **15** mins

2 **parsnips** (about 350 g/12 oz), peeled and cut into 1 cm/1/2 inch cubes

150–175 ml/5–6 fl oz **baby's usual milk**

Steam or boil the parsnips in a saucepan over a medium heat for 10–12 minutes until very tender. Puree the parsnips with the milk in a food processor, or using a hand blender, until smooth.

butternut squash

makes **30** spoons cook **15** mins

1/2 **butternut squash** (about 250 g/ 9 oz), peeled

4–5 tablespoons **baby's usual milk**

Cut the squash in half and scoop out the seeds. Cut the flesh into 1 cm/ 1/2 inch cubes. Steam or boil the squash in a saucepan over a medium heat for 15 minutes or until very tender. Puree the squash with the milk in a food processor, or using a hand blender, until smooth.

swede

makes **30** spoons cook **20** mins

1/2 **swede** (about 250 g/9 oz), peeled and cut into 1 cm/1/2 inch cubes

4–5 tablespoons **baby's usual milk**

Steam or boil the swede in a saucepan over a medium heat for 20 minutes or until completely tender. Puree the swede with the milk in a food processor, or using a hand blender, until smooth.

brussels sprouts

makes **30** spoons cook **15** mins

150 g/51/2 oz **Brussels sprouts**

4–5 tablespoons **baby's usual milk**

Cut off the base of the sprouts and remove the outer leaves. Cut the sprouts in halves or quarters and steam in a saucepan over a medium heat for 10–12 minutes until very tender (steaming is best, as boiled sprouts can taste bitter). Puree the sprouts with the milk in a food processor, or using a hand blender, until smooth.

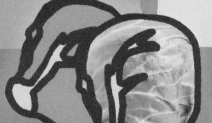

week 2 + beyond!

Now that your little one has started their foodie journey, you can begin to combine familiar tastes and introduce new food groups. Continue to offer single veg either as purees or finger food. Our planner (opposite) gives you lots of ideas! All the recipes in this chapter are not only new taste experiences but they start to work in vital nutrients, too.

what to give

Your baby's usual milk still provides their main source of nutrition so keep feeding on demand. Once your little one is munching on a range of foods at one or more meals a day, you might find they start to want less milk but make sure you still offer around 600 ml/20 fl oz of their usual milk a day.

By the age of 6 months, babies' natural iron stores are beginning to run low so it's important to offer iron-rich foods such as green veg, pulses (like lentils) and red meat. Vitamin C helps little ones absorb plant-based iron so try combining iron-rich foods with citrus fruits (take a peek at our Lentils, Squash, Orange + Tomato on page 42).

If you're offering purees, you can start to combine all the yummy veg that your baby has already tasted, as well as introduce fruit, pulses, grains (like oats) and introduce allergen foods like milk or wheat (see pages 22–24 for advice on introducing allergens). Dairy foods such as full-fat yogurts, fromage frais and cheese provide calcium for growing bones (but don't give cows' milk as a drink just yet as it won't offer the right nutrients for your baby to grow and develop compared with their usual milk).

Pulses, eggs and dairy provide protein power for growing little bodies and, once you've introduced these, you can start to add in small amounts of meat and fish if you wish.

As weaning progresses, try to pop a protein food into one and then two meals a day, alongside a carbohydrate food and one or two fruits or veggies, plus a dairy food, or alternative.

tips on texture

Once little ones are used to swallowing a thin puree, usually after a week or two, you can start to offer a thicker but still smooth texture. Just use a bit less liquid when diluting the puree or add a little baby rice so you end up with a texture like mashed potato. The puree should hold its shape when on a spoon but plop off easily if you give the spoon a flick. Avoid anything with a sticky or firm texture though.

Finger foods should still be super-melty and squish easily between your thumb and finger. Keep them in sticks the size and shape of your index finger. At this stage, you might find it easier to introduce meat and pulses in puree form as the textures can be too lumpy, stringy or firm for little ones who aren't used to chewing.

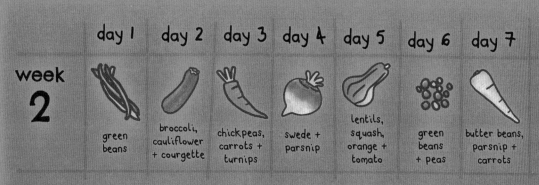

week 2	day 1	day 2	day 3	day 4	day 5	day 6	day 7
	green beans	broccoli, cauliflower + courgette	chickpeas, carrots + turnips	swede + parsnip	lentils, squash, orange + tomato	green beans + peas	butter beans, parsnip + carrots

Try 1–2 spoonfuls just after lunchtime milk (or whatever time suits you and your baby best!), building up day by day, led by your baby's appetite.

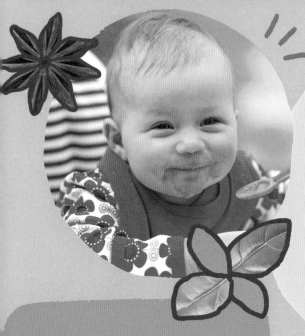

tingling taste buds

Don't feel you have to offer only bland tastes just because your baby is experiencing food for the first time. Sprinkle different spices and herbs into your baby's food for a taste adventure. Make sure you heat dried herbs through completely, puree and don't leave any woody bits.

Don't forget a rainbow of veg and fruit, a variety of grains and different protein foods from pulses and dairy to meat and fish, too!

how much?

Even though little ones grow quickly, their tummies are still teeny tiny (about the size of their clenched fist). Slowly build up the amount of food you offer at one meal, once a day, paying attention to their appetite. Watch out for the signs that your little one has had enough (see page 17).

diluting purees

Many of the recipes in this chapter suggest diluting with your baby's usual milk. This adds nutrients as well as a familiar taste but you can use the cooking water or boiled water instead, if you prefer.

41

lentils, squash, orange + tomato

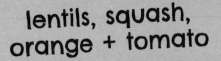

 makes **14** ice cubes prep **10** mins cook **20** mins

40 g/1½ oz dried split **red lentils**, rinsed

60 g/2¼ oz **butternut squash**, peeled, deseeded and cubed

1 **tomato**, deseeded and diced

4 tablespoons fresh **orange juice**

Place the lentils and squash in a saucepan, cover with water and bring to the boil, then reduce the heat and simmer for 10 minutes, skimming off any foam. Add the tomato and cook for a further 5 minutes or until everything is tender, then drain.

Puree the lentils, squash and tomato with the orange juice in a food processor, or using a hand blender, until smooth.

leek, cheese + potato

 makes **18** ice cubes prep **10** mins cook **25** mins

1 tablespoon **olive oil**

1 **leek**, trimmed, cleaned and chopped

1 **potato** (about 200 g/7 oz), peeled and diced

1 teaspoon **thyme leaves**

10 g/½ oz **mature Cheddar cheese**, finely grated

6–7 tablespoons **baby's usual milk**

Heat the oil in a saucepan over a low heat and cook the leek for 5 minutes until softened. Add the potato and thyme, cover with water and bring to the boil, then reduce the heat and simmer for 15 minutes or until the potato is tender. Drain.

Puree the vegetables with the cheese and the milk in a food processor, or using a hand blender, until smooth. For a smoother puree, pass it through a sieve after blending.

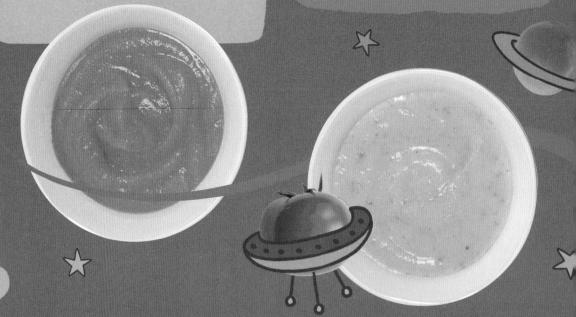

green beans + peas

makes 8 ice cubes **prep** 5 mins **cook** 10 mins

100 g/3½ oz **green beans**, trimmed and halved

100 g/3½ oz **frozen peas**

100 ml/3½ fl oz **baby's usual milk**

Steam or boil the beans in a saucepan over a medium heat for 3 minutes. Add the peas and cook for a further 2–3 minutes until the vegetables are tender.

Puree the vegetables with the milk in a food processor, or using a hand blender, until the peas are completely broken down and the mixture is smooth. For a smoother puree, pass it through a sieve after blending.

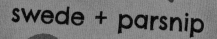

swede + parsnip

makes 13 ice cubes **prep** 5 mins **cook** 20 mins

½ **swede** (about 100 g/3½ oz), peeled and diced

1 small **parsnip** (about 75 g/2½ oz), peeled and diced

5 tablespoons **baby's usual milk**

Steam or boil the swede in a saucepan over a medium heat for 15 minutes.

Add the parsnip and cook for a further 5 minutes or until tender. Puree with the milk in a food processor, or using a hand blender, until smooth.

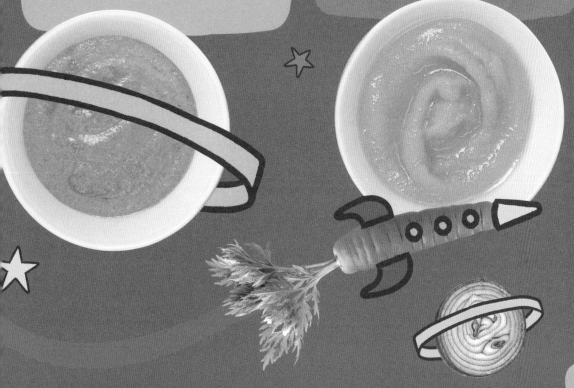

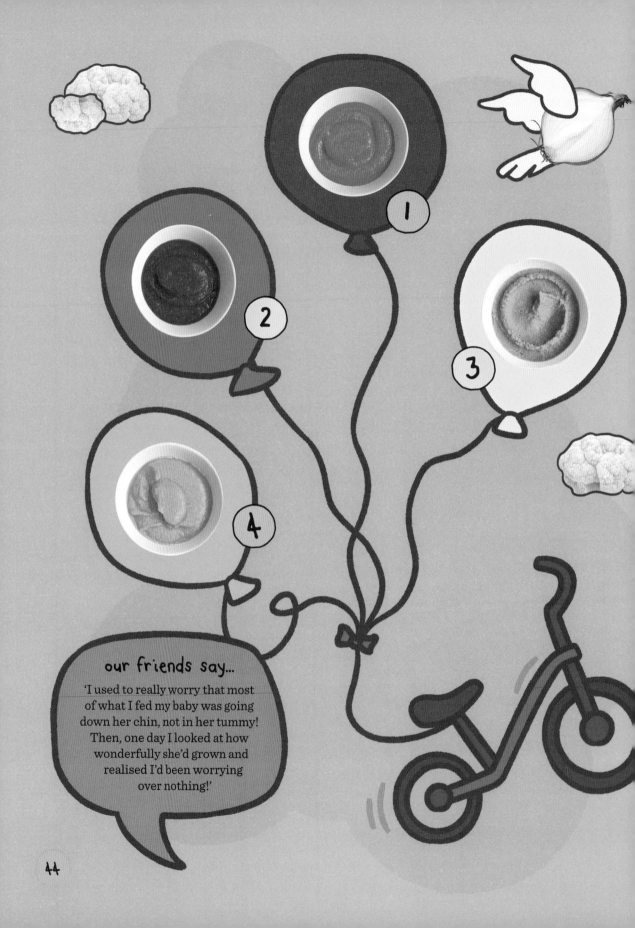

our friends say...

'I used to really worry that most of what I fed my baby was going down her chin, not in her tummy! Then, one day I looked at how wonderfully she'd grown and realised I'd been worrying over nothing!'

1 sweet potato + red pepper

 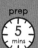

makes	prep	cook
17 ice cubes	5 mins	15 mins

1 **sweet potato** (about 250 g/9 oz), peeled and cubed

1/2 small **red pepper**, deseeded and chopped

3–4 tablespoons **baby's usual milk**

In a saucepan, steam or boil the sweet potato for 5 minutes. Add the pepper and cook for 10 minutes or until the potatoes are tender. In a food processor or using a hand blender, puree with the milk until smooth.

2 red cabbage + apples

makes	prep	cook
12 ice cubes	10 mins	20 mins

1/4 **red cabbage** (about 70 g/2 1/2 oz), finely chopped

2 eating **apples**, peeled, cored and cut into bite-sized pieces

2–3 tablespoons **baby's usual milk**

Put the cabbage and apples in a saucepan. Pour in 125 ml/4 fl oz water, cover with a lid and bring almost to boiling point over a medium heat. Reduce the heat to low and simmer for 15–18 minutes until everything is very tender. In a food processor or using a hand blender, puree with the milk until smooth.

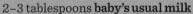

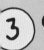

3 cauliflower, pepper, spinach + couscous

makes	prep	cook
22 ice cubes	5 mins	15 mins

100 g/3 1/2 oz **couscous**

120 g/4 1/4 oz **cauliflower**, cut into florets

1/2 **yellow pepper** (about 80 g/2 3/4 oz), cored, deseeded and diced

Large handful (about 20 g/3/4 oz) **spinach**

1 heaped teaspoon **cashew butter**

Cook the couscous according to the packet instructions. Steam or boil the cauliflower and pepper in a saucepan over a medium heat for 10 minutes or until tender. Add the spinach and cook for 1 minute or until wilted. While still warm, add the cashew butter. Leave to cool and then chill in the fridge for 40 minutes. Puree with the couscous until smooth.

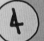

4 butternut squash, sweetcorn + peas

makes	prep	cook
21 ice cubes	10 mins	15 mins

1/2 **butternut squash** (about 400 g/14 oz), peeled, deseeded and cubed

100 g/3 1/2 oz drained no-salt, no-sugar canned **sweetcorn**

60 g/2 1/4 oz **frozen peas**

5 tablespoons **baby's usual milk**

Steam or boil the squash in a saucepan over a medium heat for 10 minutes. Add the sweetcorn and peas and cook for 5 minutes more or until everything is tender. Puree with the milk until smooth.

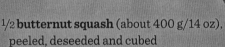

chickpeas, carrots + sweetcorn

makes	prep	cook
22 ice cubes	**5** mins	**10** mins

2 **carrots** (about 150 g/5½ oz), peeled and thinly sliced

120 g/4¼ oz) drained canned **chickpeas** in water, rinsed

100 g/3½ oz drained no-salt, no-sugar canned **sweetcorn**, saving 50 ml/2 fl oz sweetcorn water from the can

Steam or boil the carrots in a saucepan over a medium heat for 10 minutes or until tender. Puree the carrots with the chickpeas, sweetcorn and sweetcorn water in a food processor, or using a hand blender, until smooth.

peas, courgette, mint + rice

makes	prep	cook
8 ice cubes	**5** mins	**15** mins

25 g/1 oz white **basmati rice**

1 **courgette** (about 150 g/5½ oz), diced

40 g/1½ oz **frozen peas**

4 **mint leaves**

2 tablespoons **baby's usual milk**

Cook the rice according to the packet instructions until tender. Meanwhile, steam or boil the courgette over a medium heat for 5 minutes. Add the peas and cook for a further 3 minutes until the vegetables are tender. Puree the vegetables with the cooked rice, mint and the milk in a food processor, or using a hand blender, until the mixture is smooth. For a smoother puree, pass it through a sieve after blending.

swede, carrots + cinnamon

makes	prep	cook
30 ice cubes	**5** mins	**20** mins

⅓ **swede** (about 175 g/6 oz), peeled and diced

2 **carrots** (about 150 g/5½ oz), peeled and thinly sliced

Generous pinch of **ground cinnamon**

125 ml/4 fl oz **baby's usual milk**

Steam or boil the swede in a saucepan over a medium heat for 10 minutes. Add the carrots and cook for a further 10 minutes or until the veg is tender. Puree with the cinnamon and the milk in a food processor, or using a hand blender, until smooth.

pear + avocado

serves	prep	cook
1	**10** mins	no cook

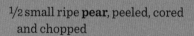

½ small ripe **pear**, peeled, cored and chopped

½ small ripe **avocado**, peeled, stoned and chopped

2 tablespoons **natural yogurt** or **baby's usual milk**, plus extra if needed

Squeeze of **lemon juice**

Puree the pear, avocado, yogurt or milk and lemon juice in a food processor, or using a hand blender, until smooth, adding a little extra yogurt or milk if necessary.

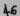

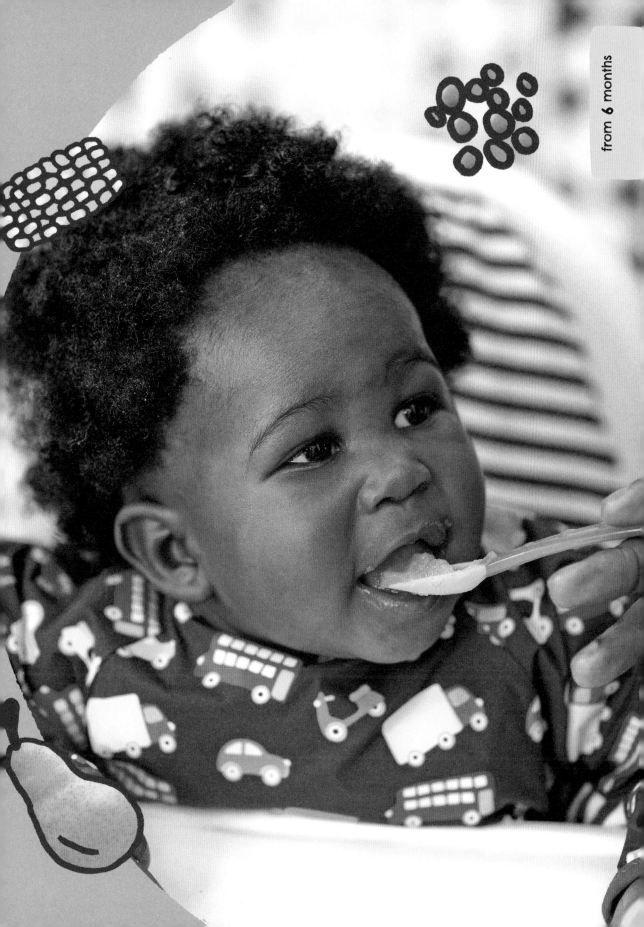

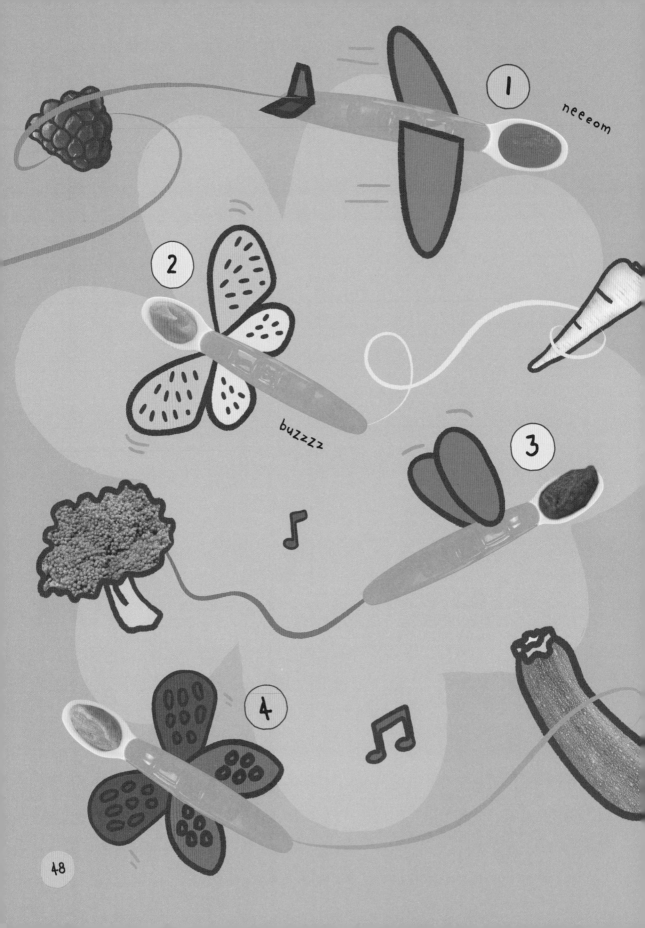

neeeom

buzzzz

48

1. papaya + raspberries

   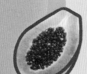

makes 2 ice cubes | **prep** 10 mins | **cook** 10 mins

1 **papaya**, peeled, deseeded and diced

70 g/2½ oz **raspberries**

Puree the papaya and raspberries in a food processor, or using a hand blender, until smooth.

2. butter beans, parsnip + carrots

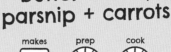

makes 2 ice cubes | **prep** 10 mins | **cook** 10 mins

1 **parsnip** (about 150 g/5½ oz), peeled

2 **carrots** (about 150 g/5½ oz), peeled and thinly sliced

100 g/3½ oz drained canned **butter beans** in water, rinsed

6 tablespoons **baby's usual milk**

Steam or boil the parsnip and carrots in a saucepan over a medium heat for 10–12 minutes until tender. Puree with the beans and the milk in a food processor, or using a hand blender, until smooth.

3. butternut squash, broccoli, beef + tomatoes

      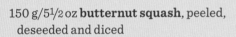

makes 2 ice cubes | **prep** 10 mins | **cook** 10 mins

150 g/5½ oz **butternut squash**, peeled, deseeded and diced

½ small head **broccoli** (about 90 g/3¼ oz), cut into small florets

80 g/2¾ oz **minced beef**

Olive oil, for cooking

100 g/3½ oz canned **chopped tomatoes**

2 tablespoons **baby's usual milk**

Steam or boil the squash in a saucepan over a medium heat for 5 minutes. Add the broccoli and cook for a further 5 minutes or until all the vegetables are tender. Meanwhile, pan-fry the beef in a little oil over a medium heat until thoroughly cooked. Puree the vegetables with the cooked beef, tomatoes and the milk in a food processor, or using a hand blender, until smooth.

4. chickpeas, courgette, carrot + coriander

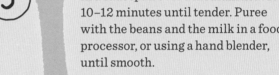   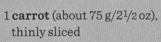 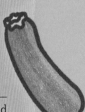

makes 2 ice cubes | **prep** 10 mins | **cook** 10 mins

1 **carrot** (about 75 g/2½ oz), thinly sliced

1 **courgette** (about 100 g/3½ oz), diced

100 g/3½ oz canned **chickpeas**, rinsed

10 fresh **coriander leaves**

3–4 tablespoons **baby's usual milk**

Steam or boil the carrot and courgette in a saucepan over a medium heat for 8–10 minutes until tender. Add the coriander leaves and heat through. Puree with the chickpeas and the milk until smooth.

broccoli, cauliflower + courgette

1

makes 15 ice cubes | **prep** 10 mins | **cook** 10 mins

1/2 small head **broccoli** (about 150 g/ 5 1/2 oz), cut into small florets

1/3 small head **cauliflower** (about 150 g/ 5 1/2 oz), cut into small florets

1 **courgette** (about 150 g/5 1/2 oz), diced

1 teaspoon chopped **parsley**

3–4 tablespoons **baby's usual milk**

Steam or boil the vegetables in a saucepan over a medium heat for 7–8 minutes until tender. Add the parsley and heat through. Puree with the milk in a food processor, or using a hand blender, until smooth.

peaches + blueberries

2

makes 5 ice cubes | **prep** 5 mins | **cook** no cook

3 ripe **peaches**, halved, stoned and diced

80 g/2 3/4 oz **blueberries**

3 tablespoons **baby's usual milk**

Puree the peaches and blueberries with the milk in a food processor, or using a hand blender, until all the fruit skin is broken down and the mixture is smooth.

oats, banana + mixed spice

3

makes 12 ice cubes | **prep** 5 mins | **cook** 10 mins

25 g/1 oz **porridge oats**

200 ml/7 fl oz **baby's usual milk**, plus extra if needed

Large pinch of ground **mixed spice**

1 small ripe **banana**, sliced

Place the oats, milk and mixed spice in a small saucepan and bring to the boil, then reduce to a simmer for 8–10 minutes, stirring frequently, until the oats are soft. Puree with the banana in a food processor, or using a hand blender, until smooth, adding extra milk if necessary.

sweet potato, carrot, broccoli + turkey

4

makes 24 ice cubes | **prep** 10 mins | **cook** 15 mins

1 small **sweet potato** (about 150 g/5 1/2 oz), peeled and diced

1 small **carrot** (about 80 g/2 3/4 oz), peeled and thinly sliced

1/4 small head **broccoli** (about 90 g/ 3 1/4 oz), cut into small florets

60 g/2 1/4 oz **minced turkey**

Olive oil, for cooking

2 tablespoons **baby's usual milk**

Steam or boil the sweet potato for 5 minutes. Add the carrot and cook for 5 minutes more, then add the broccoli and cook for a further 5 minutes or until the veg is tender. Pan-fry the turkey in a little oil over a medium heat until cooked through. Puree the veg with the turkey and milk until smooth.

2 peaches + blueberries

1 broccoli, cauliflower + courgette

3 oats, banana + mixed spice

4 sweet potato, carrot, broccoli + turkey

three ways with no-cook purees

Sometimes it helps to have a
few quick-and-easy, no-cook purees
up your sleeve for when time is short.
All of these can be rustled up in minutes and
will make one hungry-baby portion. And just for
fun, for each baby puree we've given a grown-up
or toddler variation, too. Something for everyone!

1 multi-melons + banana

what you need

75 g/2½ oz **watermelon** flesh,
deseeded and diced

75 g/2½ oz **gala or cantaloupe
melon** flesh, diced

1 small **banana**

1 tablespoon **natural Greek
yogurt** (optional)

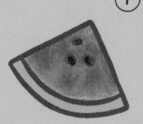

what to do

1   Put the melon and banana into a
small bowl and whiz using a hand
blender until completely smooth,
then stir in the yogurt (if using). Pass
the puree through a sieve to remove
any stringy pieces, if needed.

just for older ones

Double the recipe and take out your baby's
portion. Pour 100 ml/3½ fl oz fresh apple
juice into the remainder and whiz again.
Serve over ice with a straw for a perfect
summertime smoothie.

our friends say...

'My baby and I were so often out
and about, I created an on-the-go
feeding survival kit! It had bowls with
clip-top lids for puree, a little cool
bag with squidgy freezer packs and
plenty of spoons in case any
went on the floor!'

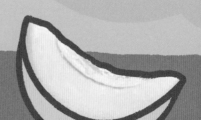

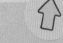

2 peach + cucumber cream

what you need

1 ripe **peach**, peeled and stoned, or 1/2 small can peach slices in juice

2.5 cm/1 inch piece of **cucumber**, peeled and deseeded

1 tablespoon natural **Greek yogurt**

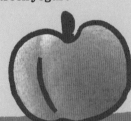

what to do

1. Chop the peach flesh and put it in a small bowl with the cucumber. Whiz using a hand blender until completely smooth. Add the Greek yogurt and stir to completely combine.

just for older ones

Double the recipe and take out your baby's portion. To the remainder, add an extra tablespoon of yogurt and spoon into a ramekin. Sprinkle with granola and serve it up for a yummy breakfast or dessert.

3 tangy kiwi + avocado

what you need

1 **kiwi fruit**

1/2 **avocado**, peeled, stoned and chopped

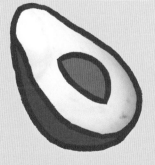

what to do

1. Peel the kiwi and chop the flesh. Put the flesh in a bowl with the avocado. Whiz using a hand blender until completely smooth. Pass through a sieve to remove any remaining kiwi pips, if you like (although the pips are tiny and will be fine for little ones over 7 months of age). Serve immediately.

just for older ones

If you want to use up the whole of the avocado, double the recipe, then take out what your baby needs. To the remainder, add a squeeze of lemon juice and a splosh of olive oil, whiz it up and drizzle it over a green salad – delicious!

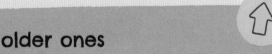

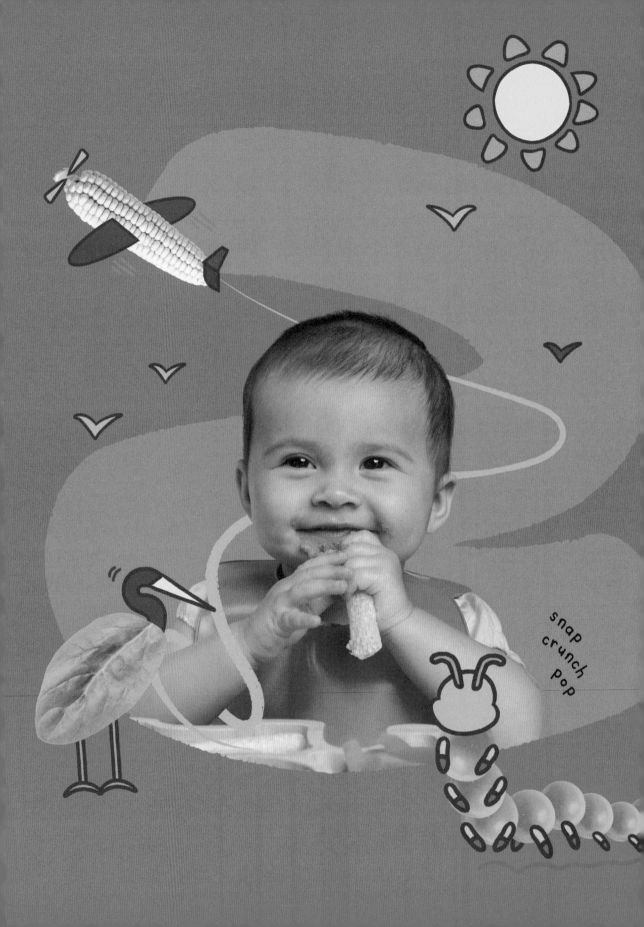

snap
crunch
pop

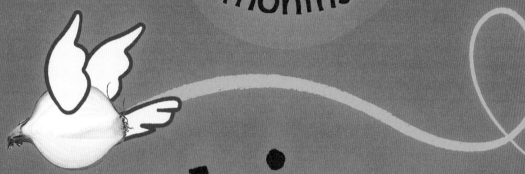

taking on texture

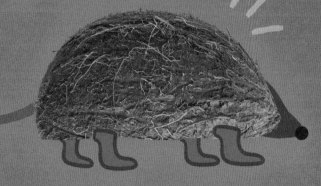

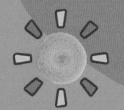

from 7 months

Your baby will probably have got the hang of eating a range of foods by now + will be developing more of an appetite! Now's the time for even more exciting tastes as well as textures. The recipes in this chapter have been created as complete meals so you can be sure you're offering variety + balance to your little one.

what to give

Food is now delivering important nutrients as well as exciting new tastes so it's super important to offer plenty of deeelicious variety and balanced meals, alongside around 600 ml/20 fl oz of your baby's usual milk each day.

Try combining the following food groups when making meals:

☺ Carbohydrate foods such as potatoes, rice, pasta, bread, oats and other grains. These provide B vitamins for energy release and fibre.

☺ Protein foods like pulses, fish, meat, egg and tofu. They can help little bones and muscles to grow and provide minerals like iron and zinc, which support the immune system.

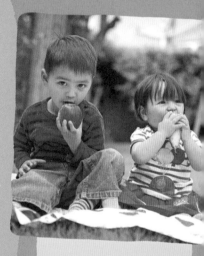

☺ Vegetables or fruits in a rainbow of colours, which provide vitamins, minerals and fibre. The more colour variety the better!

☺ Dairy foods like yogurt and cheese (or dairy-free alternatives, if you prefer, fortified with calcium, iodine and vitamins D and B12). They provide calcium to support growing bones as well as iodine, which helps little bodies grow. Check out our recipes for Yummy Yogurt Pots, Easy-cheesy-eggy Bread and Fin-tastic Little Fishy Pie (see pages 64, 66 and 78).

You can also include sources of essential fats in some meals, for example, avocado, olive or rapeseed oil, oily fish and nut and seed butters. Some of these fats, like omega-3s, can help support brain and eye development, especially those from oily fish like salmon (see pages 78, 93, 121 and 129), mackerel (see page 167) and sardines (see page 120), as well as walnuts (but they need to be finely ground).

tingling taste buds

Little ones are very open-minded so you don't need to stick to bland foods. Give some spices with a bit of oomph, such as curry powder (see page 89 – My First Chicken Curry) and cinnamon (see page 86 – Poppin' in-a-pot Wonder!).

tips on texture

By this age, your baby can start to move food from side to side in their mouth as well as use their tongue to mush small soft lumps against the roof of their mouth with an up and down movement. They can also grasp stick-like objects in their hand, using their thumb for balance, so they are getting better at holding finger foods as well as munching more textured food.

Instead of blending purees till they are smooth, you can blitz food more coarsely or mash with a fork to achieve a thicker texture with small soft lumps (smaller than a lentil) in a thick puree that holds its shape on a spoon. Even if little ones don't have teeth, they can still mush those tiny lumps with their tongue and giving them more textured food helps them develop chewing skills.

Avoid whole peas and sweetcorn, stringy or gristly meat and hard pasta as these can pose a choking risk. And it's best to puree foods with tough skins or a stringy texture like peppers, celery, green beans, pulses and onions.

Offer finger foods at each meal to help your little one develop hand-eye coordination. As well as cooked veg and soft fruit, you can try bread or toast fingers and well-cooked pasta pieces (penne is easy to hold), all still the shape and size of your index finger. Finger foods should still be super soft, melty and squishable between your thumb and finger. For a great finger food breakfast idea, check out our recipe for Three Ways with Pancakes on pages 68–69!

nutritionist know-how

Textured food and finger food not only help little ones to learn to chew – they also help them to develop those little mouth muscles, encouraging speech development.

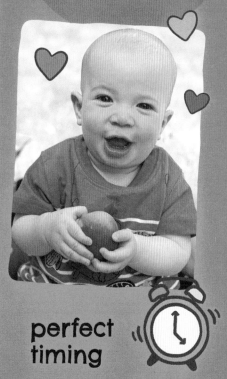

how much?

Little ones are really good at knowing when they've had enough to eat, so be led by them and let your baby tell you when enough is enough. (For signs they're full, see page 17.) Some days your baby won't fancy much food, while on others they'll be super hungry so be responsive to their appetite. Try not to worry – it's what they eat over a week or more that counts so don't be concerned by the odd off day or two.

perfect timing

Once your little one is happy gobbling up a decent serving once a day, you can introduce a second and then a third meal. If they're having a good lunch then maybe try offering breakfast or dinner as well, whichever works for you and your baby! Aim for your baby to be having three meals a day by the time they are 7 or 8 months old but go at your own pace as every baby is different.

three ways with
Ella's Kitchen friends

We think the best weaning advice of all is passed on by word of mouth – from parents + grandparents, aunts + uncles, and from one friend to another. Some of those nuggets of wisdom might strike a chord + fire up an idea, others might reassure you or make you smile + know that you aren't alone. We've asked some of our Ella's Kitchen Friends for the best pieces of weaning advice others had given them.

These are the ones we especially hope will inspire you to relax + enjoy this special time with your baby.

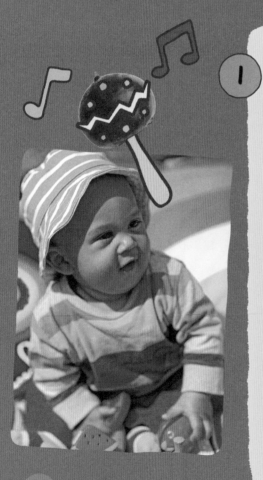

1 stick up lists

When I started weaning my little girl, the best piece of advice I think anyone ever gave me was to stick up a step-by-step list of when to introduce certain foods.

It was a simple idea, but it made a big difference to us. It simplified the weaning process, which initially felt quite daunting. Once it was up, that list meant I could look on the fridge and plan my shopping with my baby in mind, knowing everything I bought for her was safe and providing the right nutrients.

It also made it exciting when it was time to introduce something new – we'd celebrate with lots of smiles and cries of 'Well done!' Everyone was happy!

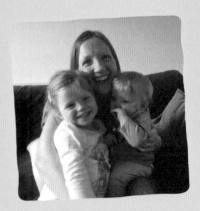

Saffron, mum to Allana (age 3) and Iris (age 8 months)

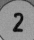

2

look at a week

I used to think my little one was such a fussy eater and that he wasn't eating enough. Then, my health visitor told me I shouldn't think of his diet as something that happens over a day, but over the course of a week, or even a month. That was my lightbulb moment!

It sounds a bit grown-up, but I kept a food diary of everything he ate and the amount of time he spent breastfeeding every day for a month. It was amazing to see that some days he ate precious little in the way of food, but he certainly made up for it on others! Seeing everything written down made me realize that over a whole week, and then a whole month, he was eating perfectly well and getting everything he needed – he was just doing it his own special way!

Angie, mum to Reece (age 5) and Summer (age 2)

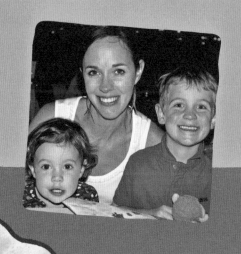

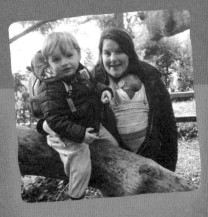

3

turn the table

My baby boy was absolutely brilliant at eating in his high chair in the early days, but when he got a bit more mobile, he started objecting to sitting at the table. He wanted to eat on the move all the time!

My dad told me not to let it become a battle (eventually he'd sit where the rest of us were sitting), and to think of 'creative' tables around our home. At teatime, I took to laying out a picnic rug on the kitchen floor, with a few teddies, too; on warm days, we'd picnic in the garden. Teatimes were so much more relaxed this way that eventually, after only a couple of weeks and without him even really noticing, he was back in his high chair and eating at the table happily.

Occasionally – even though he's now 3 – we still have an indoor picnic...just for fun!

Sophie, mum to Tristan (age 3) and Alice (age 10 months)

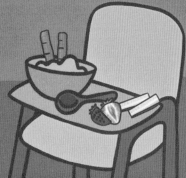

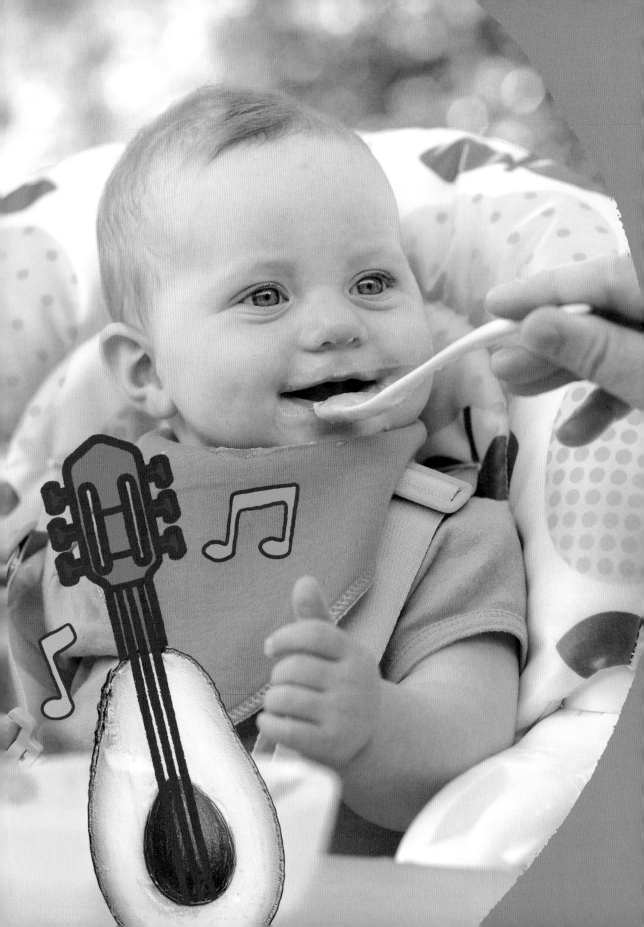

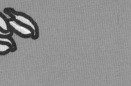
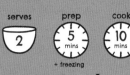

serves **2**

prep **5** mins

cook **10** mins

+ freezing

bright starts brekkie bowl

We've given smoothies a veggie shake-up! Perfect for hot summer days, this cool + creamy brekkie bowl is a great way to get your little one to eat more veg.

what you need

1 **banana**, peeled, cut into thirds and frozen

2 **broccoli** florets (about 40 g/1½ oz)

1 tablespoon **rolled oats**

1½–2 tablespoons **whole milk or milk of choice**, plus extra if needed

1 ripe baby **avocado**, halved, stoned and flesh scooped out

¼ teaspoon **ground cinnamon**

Lightly toasted **bread**, buttered and cut into fingers, to serve

what to do

1. Take the banana out of the freezer to soften slightly while you prepare the rest of the ingredients.

2. Meanwhile, steam the broccoli in a saucepan over a medium heat for 8 minutes or until the florets are tender (you can also cook them in a microwave or an air fryer). Place under cold running water until cold.

3. Place the oats in a food processor or blender and blitz to a powder, then pour in the milk. Next, add the softened banana, avocado, cinnamon and cooked broccoli. Blend until smooth and creamy, adding a splash more milk if needed – it should have the consistency of a very thick milkshake. Spoon the mixture into bowls and serve with fingers of lightly toasted bread for dunking.

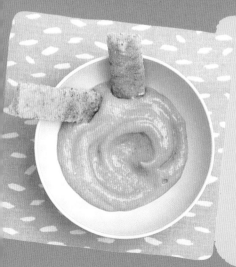

top tip!

This recipe can easily be adapted to suit your baby's favourite tastes. Here are a few quick ideas:

☺ Stir in 1 teaspoon smooth peanut butter (if your little one has already tried peanuts and had no reaction) and 1 teaspoon mixed ground seeds with the avocado and the rest of the ingredients.

☺ For little ones over 1 year, scatter your choice of finely chopped nuts and seeds over the top for a bit of crunch.

totally tropical fruity couscous

serves **2**

prep **5** mins

cook **20** mins

+ overnight defrosting

what you need

25 g/1 oz **couscous**, rinsed well

1 tablespoon **whole milk or milk of choice**

165 g/5¾ oz frozen **tropical fruit mix**, defrosted overnight in the fridge

4 tablespoons **coconut milk**, the creamy part from the top of the can

2 teaspoons **ground almonds or ground mixed seeds** (optional)

what to do

1. Put the couscous in a small saucepan, pour over enough water to cover and bring to the boil, then turn the heat down and simmer, part-covered with a lid, for 20 minutes or until the grains are very tender. Drain the couscous, pour in the milk, then stir.

2. Place the defrosted tropical fruit and coconut milk in a food processor or blender and blend to a thick puree, then stir the mixture into the couscous with the ground almonds or seeds (if using). Spoon into bowls and serve.

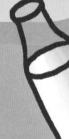

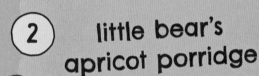

little bear's apricot porridge

serves **3–4**

prep **5** mins

cook **10** mins

+ overnight soaking

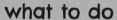

what you need

4 unsulphured, dark **dried apricots**, roughly chopped

40 g/1½ oz **porridge oats**

½ teaspoon **ground nutmeg or cinnamon**

300 ml/½ pint **baby's usual milk**, plus extra if needed

what to do

1. Put the apricots and 3 tablespoons of just-boiled water in a heatproof bowl and leave to soak overnight. The following morning, blend the apricots and their soaking water to a puree in a food processor, or using a hand blender, adding another 1 tablespoon of water if needed.

2. Place the oats, nutmeg or cinnamon and milk in a small saucepan and bring to the boil, then reduce the heat and simmer, stirring frequently, for 8 minutes or until the oats are cooked. Stir in the apricot puree and heat through briefly.

3. Using the back of a fork, mash the oat mixture until almost smooth, adding a little extra milk if necessary. Alternatively, puree in a food processor or using a hand blender.

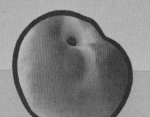

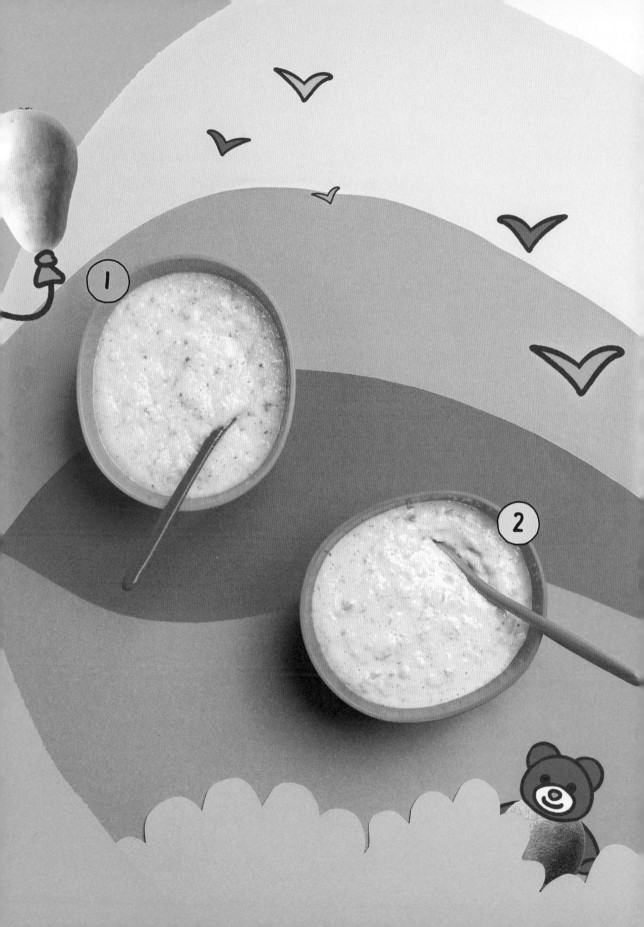

three ways with
yummy yogurt pots

Yogurt is one of our go-to, quick + easy brekkies. Here, we've pear-ed up three yummy sweet + savoury combos to get you started but feel free to get creative and mix + match your little one's favourite tastes!

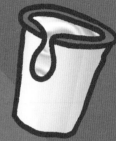

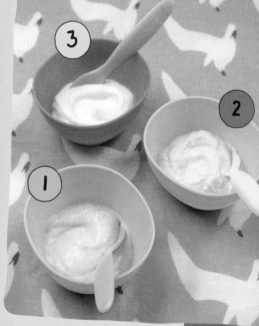

1 summery strawberries + cucumber

serves 2 | prep 5 mins | cook no cook

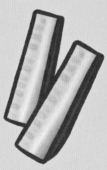

what you need

40 g/1½ oz **cucumber**, peeled and cut into chunks

8 **strawberries**, hulled

Natural Greek yogurt, to serve

what to do

1. Put the cucumber and strawberries in a food processor or blender and puree until smooth. Serve on top of or stirred into the yogurt.

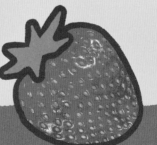

2

apple + butternut squash

serves **2** | prep **5** mins | cook **15** mins

what you need

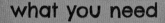

1 **eating apple**, peeled, cored, and cut into small bite-sized chunks

40 g/1½ oz **butternut squash**, peeled and cut into small bite-sized chunks

Large pinch of **mixed spice**

Natural Greek yogurt, to serve

what to do

1 Put the apple and squash in a small saucepan with 2 tablespoons of water. Place the pan over a medium–low heat and simmer, part-covered with a lid, for 12–14 minutes until the apple and squash are very soft.

2 Stir in the mixed spice and mash with the back of a fork. Alternatively, puree in a food processor or using a hand blender. Serve on top of or stirred into the yogurt.

3

pears + ginger

serves **2** | prep **5** mins | cook **10** mins (optional)

what you need

2 ripe **baby pears**, peeled and cored

Large pinch of **ground ginger**

Natural Greek yogurt, to serve

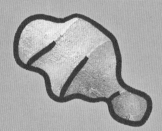

what to do

1 If the pears are very ripe, grate them into a bowl – they need to be soft, ripe and 'mashable' with the back of a fork. If the pears are slightly firm, cut them into bite-sized chunks and steam them in a saucepan over a medium heat for 8–10 minutes until very tender.

2 Stir in the ginger and mash with the back of a fork. Alternatively, puree in a food processor or using a hand blender. Serve on top of or stirred into the yogurt.

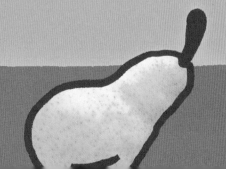

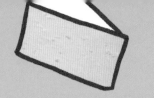

easy-cheesy-eggy bread

Try this easy-peasy cheesy eggy bread! Ready in just 15 minutes, it's perfect for big day brekkies!

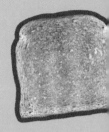

what you need

1 **egg**, lightly beaten

2 tablespoons **baby's usual milk**

10 g/¼ oz **Parmesan cheese**, finely grated

1 thick slice of **wholemeal bread**

10 g/¼ oz **unsalted butter**

what to do

1) Mix together the egg, milk and Parmesan in a shallow bowl. Add the bread and press it down lightly to immerse it in the egg mixture.

2) Heat the butter in a nonstick frying pan over a medium heat. Add the egg-soaked bread and cook for 2–3 minutes on each side until golden and slightly crisp. Cut into fingers and serve.

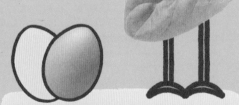

egg-cellent veggies

If you have any leftover pureed veggies, such as carrot, pea, cauliflower, broccoli or spinach, mix it into the egg mixture – about 1 tablespoon is perfect.

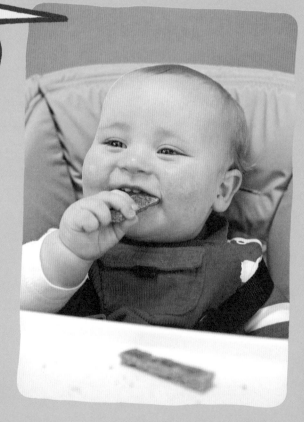

serves **1**

prep **5** mins
+ defrosting

cook **5** mins

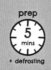

rise + shine scrambly eggs

These speedy scrambly eggs are an egg-cellent way to start the day! We've added extra greens + herbs for yummy tasty goodness. Cracked it!

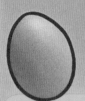

what you need

1 **egg**, lightly beaten

1 tablespoon **whole milk or milk of choice**

1/4 teaspoon **dried oregano**

5 g/1/8 oz **unsalted butter**

10 g/1/4 oz **frozen chopped spinach**, defrosted

Lightly toasted **bread**, buttered and cut into fingers, to serve

what to do

1. In a bowl, beat the egg with the milk and oregano.

2. Melt the butter in a small saucepan over a medium–low heat. Add the egg mixture to the pan and cook, stirring continuously, for 1–2 minutes until scrambled.

3. Stir in the spinach and warm through briefly. Serve the eggs with fingers of toasted bread on the side.

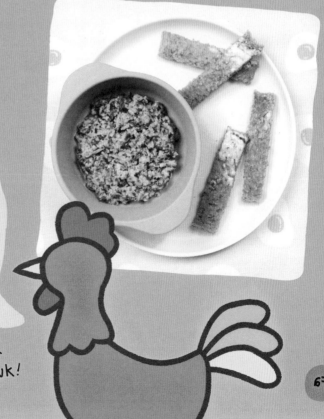

our friends say...

'It was a revelation when my health visitor told me that babies don't need teeth to eat finger foods! They can manage certain soft foods really well by mashing them between their gums as the gums harden.'

buk buk bu gawk!

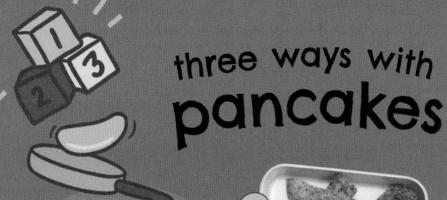

three ways with
pancakes

Rise + shine, it's pancake time! Here are three of our favourite ways to jazz up pancakes, which you can easily prepare in advance or freeze for another day. Give them a go, they're flippin' good!

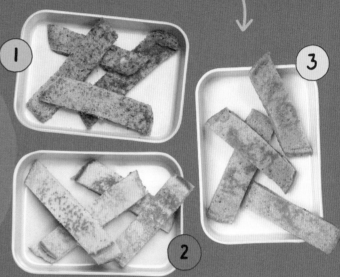

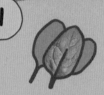

spinach, oat + cheese pancakes

 makes about **8**

 prep **5** mins

+ defrosting + resting

 cook **15** mins

what you need

50 g/1³⁄4 oz **plain flour**

50 g/1³⁄4 oz **rolled oats**

1 teaspoon **baking powder**

50 g/1³⁄4 oz **frozen chopped spinach**, defrosted

40 g/1¹⁄2 oz **mature Cheddar cheese**, grated

125 ml/4 fl oz **whole milk or milk of choice**

1 **egg**

Unsalted butter, for frying

what to do

1. Put all the ingredients, except the butter, in a food processor or blender and blend until combined. Leave the batter to rest for 20 minutes.

2. To cook the pancakes, follow the instructions in step 3 of the recipe opposite.

3. Cut the pancakes into fingers to serve.

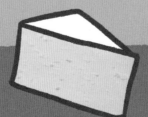

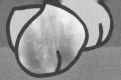

2) chickpea + corn pancakes

 makes about 8
 prep 5 mins + resting
 cook 15 mins

what you need

85 g/3 oz drained no-salt, no-sugar **canned sweetcorn**

1 **egg**

100 g/3½ oz **gram (chickpea) flour**

1 teaspoon **baking powder**

100 ml/3½ fl oz **whole milk or milk of choice**

Unsalted butter, for frying

what to do

1. Place the sweetcorn and egg in a food processor or blender and blend until almost smooth. Add the gram flour, baking powder and milk and blend again until combined. Leave the batter to rest for 20 minutes.

2. To cook the pancakes, follow the instructions in step 3 of the recipe below.

3. Cut the pancakes into fingers to serve.

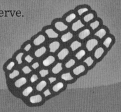

3) apple + cinnamon pancakes

 makes about 8
 prep 10 mins + resting
 cook 30 mins

what you need

2 **eating apples**, peeled, cored and cut into bite-sized pieces

100 g/3½ oz **plain flour**

1 teaspoon **baking powder**

1 **egg**

100 ml/3½ fl oz **whole milk or milk of choice**

1 teaspoon **ground cinnamon**

2 teaspoons **ground mixed seeds** (optional)

Unsalted butter, for frying

Natural Greek yogurt, to serve

what to do

1. Cook the apples with 2 tablespoons of water in a saucepan, part-covered with a lid, for 12–14 minutes until very soft. Mash with the back of a fork or puree in a food processor or using a hand blender until smooth. Leave to cool.

2. Place the flour, baking powder, egg, milk, cinnamon, mixed seeds (if using) and 85 g/3 oz of the apple puree in a food processor or blender and blend until combined. Leave the batter to rest for 20 minutes.

3. To cook the pancakes, heat a small knob of butter in a large nonstick frying pan over a medium heat. Turn the heat down a little, then add spoonfuls of the batter to the pan – about 2 tablespoons for each pancake. You should be able to fit 3 or 4 pancakes in the pan. Cook for 2 minutes on each side, turning halfway, until light golden.

4. Cut the pancakes into fingers and serve with extra apple puree and the yogurt on the side.

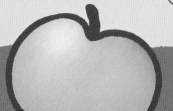

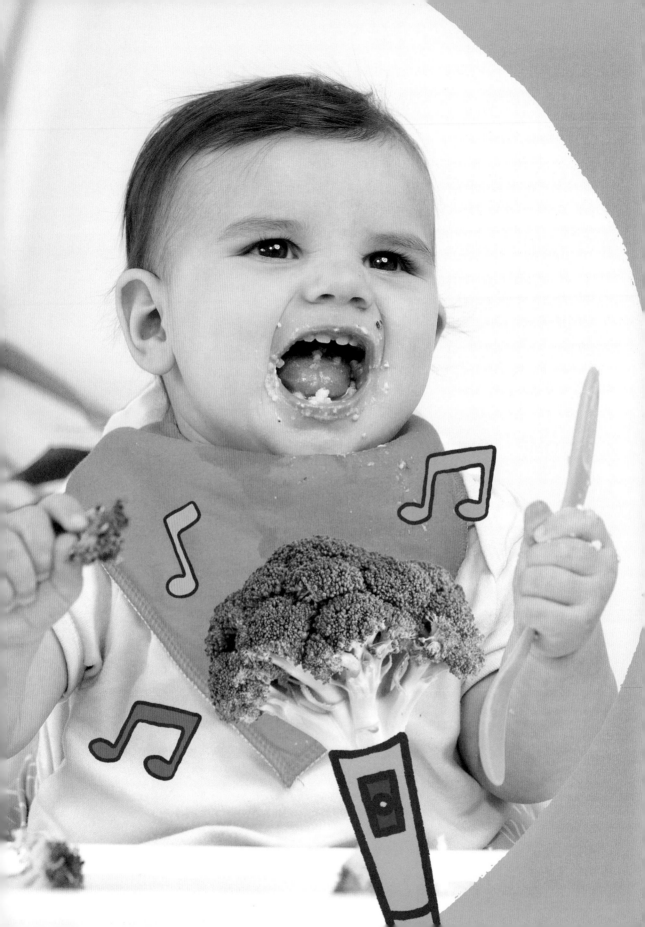

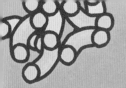

serves **2-3** · prep **5** mins · cook **10** mins

 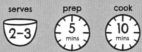

broc 'n' roll cheesy chive pasta

Ready in just 15 minutes, this cheesy chive pasta is really 'grate'. Broc 'n' roll, baby!

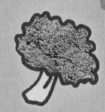

what you need

50 g/1¾ oz **dried orzo or other small pasta**

3 **broccoli florets**, cut into small pieces, plus extra, steamed until very tender, to serve

30 g/1 oz **frozen petits pois**

½ teaspoon snipped **chives**

1 tablespoon **cream cheese**

3–4 tablespoons **baby's usual milk**

what to do

1. Cook the pasta in a saucepan of boiling water for 3 minutes, then add the broccoli and petits pois and cook for a further 4–5 minutes until everything is tender. Drain, reserving the cooking water.

2. Return the pasta, vegetables and 2 tablespoons of the reserved cooking water to the pan. Add the chives, cream cheese and 3 tablespoons of the milk and warm through slightly.

3. Using the back of a fork, mash the pasta and veg mixture, making sure you crush the petits pois well, until almost smooth, adding the remaining milk if needed. Alternatively, puree using a mini food processor or hand blender. Serve in bowls with extra steamed broccoli florets as finger food.

rat-a-tat-tat!

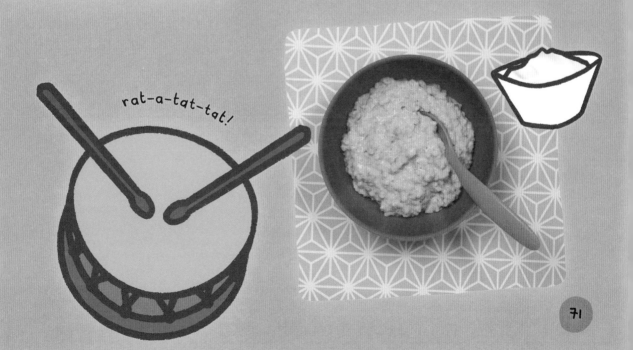

71

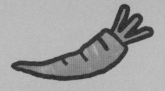

serves **3-4**
prep **10 mins**
cook **25 mins**

super-duper spaghetti + sauce!

When time is tight, give this speedy tomato pasta a go. It's packed full of store-cupboard superheroes, including lovely lentils for extra protein. Cook ahead + store in the fridge for up to two days or freeze into portions.

what you need

75 g/2½ oz **dried spaghetti**, broken into pieces

30 g/1 oz **dried split red lentils**, rinsed

1 **carrot** (about 60 g/2¼ oz), cut into batons

2 teaspoons **olive oil**

1 **garlic clove**, crushed

½ teaspoon **dried oregano**

200 ml/7 fl oz **passata** (sieved tomatoes)

2 tablespoons **whole milk or milk of choice**

Avocado slices, to serve

what to do

1. Bring a saucepan of water to the boil, then add the spaghetti pieces, lentils and carrot and cook for 12–14 minutes, or until the pasta and lentils are tender and the carrot is soft and can be squished between your fingers. Drain, reserving the cooking water.

2. Meanwhile, heat the oil in a small saucepan over a medium–low heat and cook the garlic for 1 minute, stirring. Add the oregano and passata, stir, then part-cover with a lid and simmer for 8 minutes or until the sauce has reduced and thickened.

3. Finely chop the pasta into very small pieces and mash the carrot batons with the back of a fork. Add the pasta, lentils and carrots to the sauce with the milk. Stir until combined and reheat briefly. If the texture is too coarse, mash it with the back of a fork or semi-blend in a food processor or using a hand blender, adding some of the reserved cooking water if needed.

4. Serve the pasta and sauce with the avocado slices on the side as finger food.

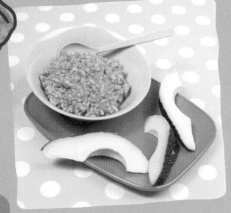

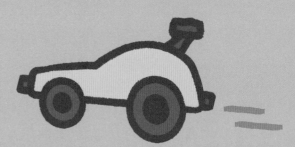

serves 1–2 | prep 10 mins | cook 15 mins

very veggie kedgeree

Start your little one off on their spice adventure with this yummy veggie kedgeree. It includes turmeric + curry powder to get their taste buds tingling! Nice 'n' not too spicy!

what you need

40 g/1½ oz **white rice**, rinsed

50 g/1¾ oz **carrot**, finely grated

50 g/1¾ oz **cauliflower florets**, finely grated

½ teaspoon **mild curry powder**

Large pinch of **ground turmeric**

1 **egg**

2 tablespoons **whole milk or milk of choice**, plus extra if needed

10 g/¼ oz **unsalted butter**

Broccoli florets, steamed until very tender, to serve

what to do

1. Put the rice, carrot, cauliflower, curry powder and turmeric in a small saucepan. Pour over enough water to cover by 1 cm/½ inch and bring to the boil. Turn the heat down to the lowest setting, cover with a lid and simmer for 12–15 minutes until the rice and vegetables are cooked and tender.

2. Meanwhile, using a fork, beat the egg with 1 tablespoon of the milk in a bowl. Heat the butter in a nonstick frying pan over a medium–low heat, add the egg mixture and cook, stirring, for 1½–2 minutes until scrambled. Spoon into a bowl and lightly mash with the back of a fork to break the scrambled egg into small pieces.

3. When the rice is cooked, stir in the remaining milk, then blend briefly with a hand blender to a coarse puree, adding a splash more milk if needed. Gently stir in the scrambled egg and serve in bowls with the steamed broccoli on the side as finger food.

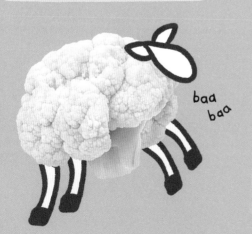

baa baa

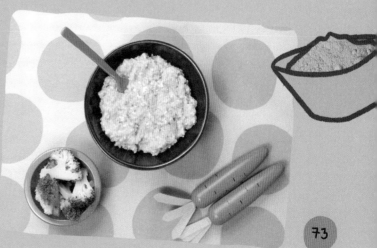

73

serves **2**
 prep **5** mins
 cook **10** mins

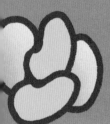

full-of-beans on toast

This tasty twist on beans on toast is made with added veg, egg + cheese. Cool beans!

what you need

1 **egg**

2 **cauliflower florets** (about 60 g/ 2¼ oz), finely grated

125 g/4½ oz drained **canned haricot beans** in water, rinsed

6 tablespoons **passata** (sieved tomatoes)

2 teaspoons **cream cheese**

Splash of **whole milk or milk of choice** (optional)

Lightly toasted **bread**, buttered and cut into fingers, to serve

what to do

1. Boil the egg in a small pan of boiling water for 8 minutes, adding the grated cauliflower 2 minutes before the end of the cooking time. Drain, leaving the cauliflower in the sieve. Cool the egg under cold running water, then peel off the shell.

2. Meanwhile, put the beans and passata in another small saucepan and simmer for 4 minutes. Stir in the cream cheese, then mash the beans with the back of a fork or roughly blend with a hand blender, if preferred.

3. Finely mash the egg with a fork, then stir it into the beans with the cauliflower, adding a splash of milk if needed. Serve with fingers of toast on the side.

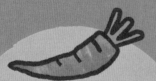

keep calm + carrot on!

If you don't have cauliflower, you can swap in cooked + finely grated carrot, butternut squash or sweet potato instead.

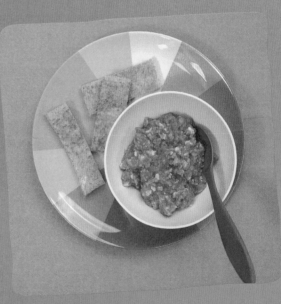

74

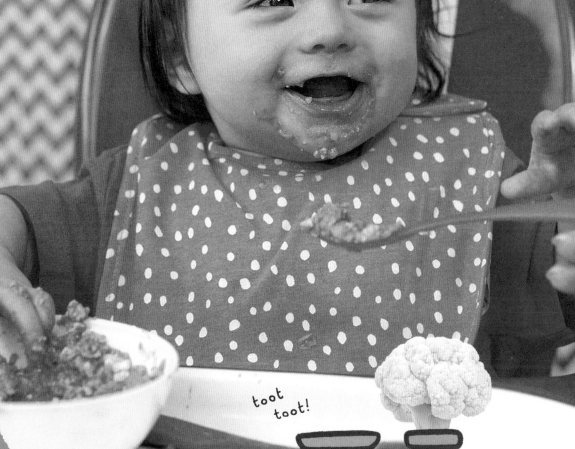

toot
toot!

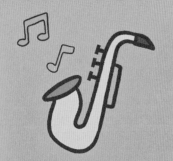

groovy veggie mash

Get into the grooooove with this yummy veggie mash. It's sure to be a mash-ed hit with your little one!

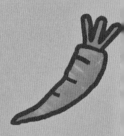

what you need

1 **carrot** (about 75 g/2¹/₂ oz), chopped into small pieces

60 g/2¹/₄ oz **white cabbage**, shredded

60 g/2¹/₄ oz **rolled oats**

300 ml/¹/₂ pint **whole milk or milk of choice**

1–1¹/₂ teaspoons no-salt, no-sugar **smooth peanut butter**

what to do

1. Steam the carrot and cabbage in a saucepan over a medium heat for 6–8 minutes until very tender.

2. Meanwhile, put the oats in a small saucepan with the milk and 100 ml/3¹/₂ fl oz of water over a medium–low heat. Bring up to bubbling point, stirring occasionally. Turn the heat down to low and simmer, stirring, for 8–10 minutes until very soft and creamy, mashing the oats down with the spoon or back of a fork.

3. Mash or blend the cooked vegetables until almost smooth, then stir them into the oats with the peanut butter (you may need to add another tablespoon of hot water) until combined.

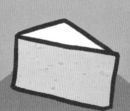

'nut' for me!

For a peanut-free alternative, stir 2 tablespoons of finely grated Cheddar cheese into the cooked oats instead.

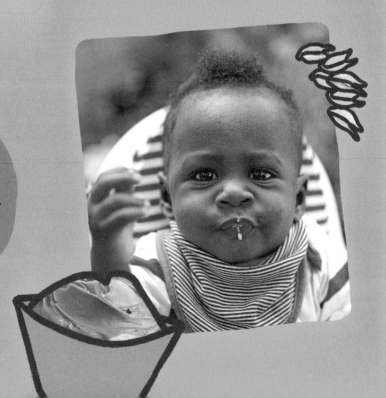

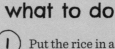

serves **2–3** prep **10 mins** cook **25 mins**

easy-pea-sy minty risotto

Risott-oh yeah! Fresh, filling + full of exciting new flavours, this recipe is just pea-fect!

what you need

50 g/1¾ oz **risotto rice**

40 g/1½ oz **frozen petits pois**

⅓ **leek**, trimmed, cleaned and finely chopped

5 **mint leaves**

1 teaspoon **unsalted butter or spread of choice**

1 tablespoon **whole milk or milk of choice**

what to do

1. Put the rice in a small saucepan and pour over 185 ml/6½ fl oz of just-boiled water. Stir the rice, then return the water to the boil. Turn the heat down to the lowest setting, cover the pan with a lid, and simmer, stirring occasionally, for 20–25 minutes until the rice is very tender and the water has been absorbed.

2. Meanwhile, steam the petits pois and leek in a saucepan over a medium heat for 4–5 minutes until soft, adding the mint leaves 1 minute before the end of the cooking time. Using a hand blender, puree the cooked vegetables and mint with the butter and milk until smooth.

3. Mash the cooked rice with the back of a fork or blend briefly with a hand blender to a coarse puree. Stir in the vegetable and mint puree.

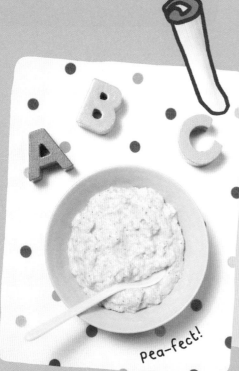

pea-fect!

herby water play

Little ones love playing with water, so how about infusing it with herby scents? Pick off a few spare mint stalks and leaves and give your little one a small bowl of water (it might be best to do this outdoors or sitting on an oilcloth on the floor). Encourage your baby to swirl and squish the leaves and stalks through the water, mixing it up really well. Now, take a little cup and scoop out some of the water. Offer it to your baby to sniff. Can you smell the herb in the water? Try with some different fresh herbs – basil, sage and rosemary work a treat.

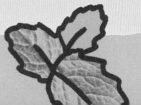

77

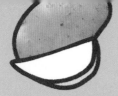

fin-tastic little fishy pie

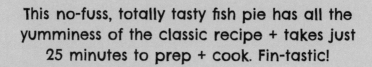

This no-fuss, totally tasty fish pie has all the yumminess of the classic recipe + takes just 25 minutes to prep + cook. Fin-tastic!

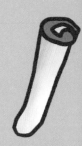

what you need

250 g/9 oz **white potatoes** for mashing, peeled and cut into small chunks

1 small **leek** (about 100 g/3½ oz), trimmed, cleaned and finely chopped

50 g/1¾ oz **frozen peas**

10 g/¼ oz **unsalted butter**

75 ml/2½ fl oz **whole milk or milk of choice**, plus extra if needed

115 g/4 oz **canned wild pink salmon or cooked pink trout or salmon fillet**, bones and skin removed, fish mashed

what to do

1. Put the potatoes in a saucepan and pour in enough water to cover. Bring to the boil and cook the potatoes for 2 minutes. Turn the heat down slightly, add the leek and peas and cook for 8 minutes or until the potatoes and vegetables are tender.

2. Drain the cooked potatoes and vegetables, then return them to the hot pan, add the butter and milk and warm through. Using a hand blender, blend the mixture to a coarse puree, adding more milk if needed.

3. Stir the mashed cooked fish into the potato mixture and serve in bowls.

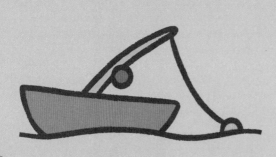

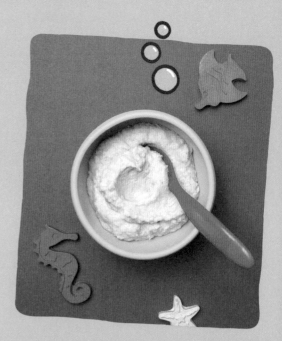

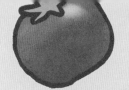

serves

2

prep

10 mins

cook

no cook

no-cook tuna + avo mash

Just right for days when time is tight, this tasty tuna mash can be ready in minutes!

what you need

1 **tomato**

1 small **avocado**, halved and stoned

Squeeze of **lemon juice**

2 tablespoons drained **canned tuna chunks** in spring water

3 tablespoons drained **canned haricot beans** in water, rinsed

Baby's usual milk (optional)

what to do

1) Place the tomato in a heatproof bowl and pour over enough just-boiled water to cover. Leave for 1–2 minutes, then carefully remove with a slotted spoon and peel off the skin. Halve the tomato, scoop out and discard the seeds, then finely chop the flesh.

2) Scoop out the avocado flesh into a bowl, squeeze over a little lemon juice and add the chopped tomato, tuna and beans. Puree using a hand blender until almost smooth, adding a little milk if necessary.

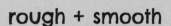
ribbet ribbet

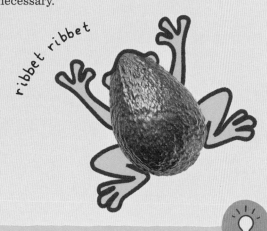

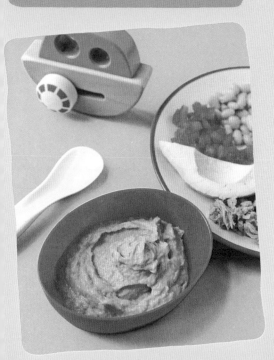

rough + smooth

A whole avocado is brilliant for teaching opposites. Let your baby feel the bumpy skin – like a crocodile! Open it up for little fingers to poke the super-smooth flesh. Talk about the textures – rough and smooth all in one!

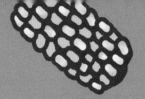

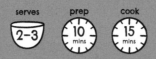

chick-chick-chicken corn chowder

Made with everyday ingredients, this
comforting chicken + corn chowder is just right
for little tums. Yuuuuuuuummmmmmm!

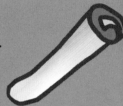

what you need

2 teaspoons **olive oil**

1 small **onion**, very finely chopped

125 g/4½ oz **minced chicken**,
   finely chopped

175 g/6 oz **potato**, peeled and cut
   into 1 cm/½ inch pieces

60 g/2¼ oz drained no-salt,
   no-sugar **canned sweetcorn**

1 small **leek**, trimmed, cleaned
   and very finely chopped

100 ml/3½ oz **whole milk or milk
of choice**, plus extra if needed

Wholemeal bread fingers,
   to serve (optional)

what to do

1. Heat the oil in a small saucepan, add the onion and minced chicken and cook over a medium heat for 5 minutes, stirring to break up the mince, until the onion has softened and the chicken is opaque.

2. Add the potato, sweetcorn, leek and 125 ml/ 4 fl oz cold water and bring to the boil. Turn the heat down to low and simmer, covered with a lid, for 5 minutes. Pour in the milk and cook for another 5 minutes or until the chicken is cooked and the vegetables are very tender.

3. Using a potato masher, mash the chicken and vegetables until almost smooth, adding a little extra hot milk or water, if necessary. Alternatively, roughly puree to a thick creamy consistency in a food processor or with a hand blender. Serve in bowls with bread fingers on the side, if liked.

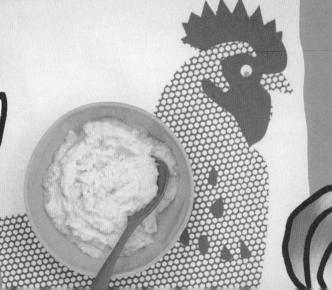

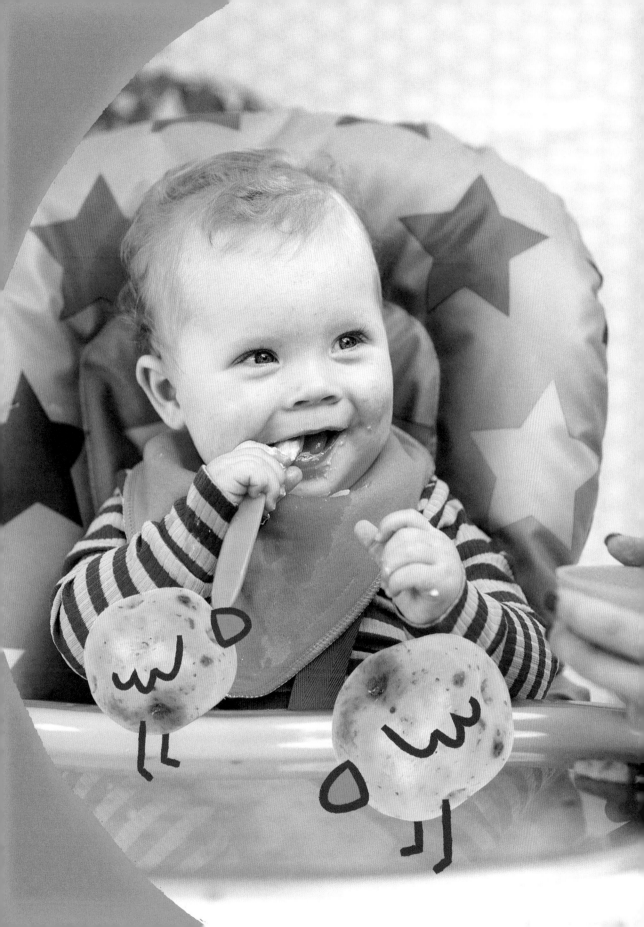

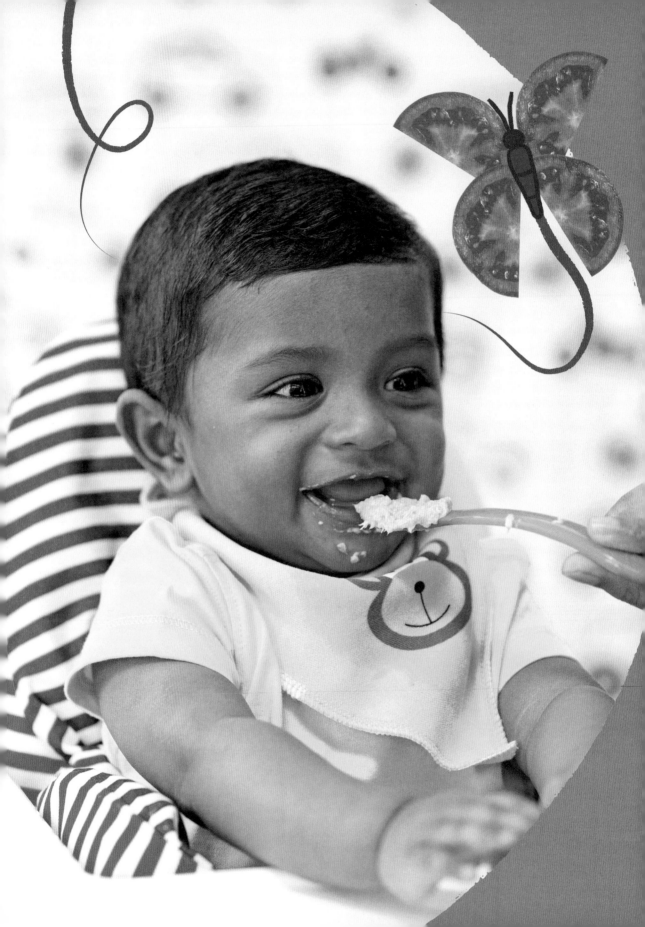

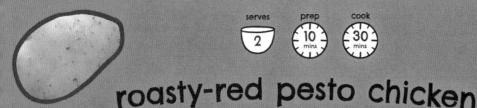

serves **2** · prep **10** mins · cook **30** mins

roasty-red pesto chicken

Juicy + textured roast chicken gives little gums that are just learning to chew a workout. With just a few ingredients, hey pesto, you're ready to go!

what you need

1 small **potato** (about 115 g/4 oz), peeled and cut into very small chunks

1 small **leek**, trimmed, cleaned and very thinly sliced

1 **tomato**, sliced into rounds

1/2 teaspoon **dried oregano**

1 teaspoon **olive oil**

1 teaspoon **red pesto** (see box, below)

1 skinless **chicken breast** (about 125 g/4 1/2 oz)

Baby's usual milk (optional)

what to do

1. Preheat the oven to 200°C/400°F/Gas Mark 6. Place a large sheet of aluminium foil in a baking dish and arrange the potato chunks in the middle in an even layer. Top with the leek and tomato, then sprinkle over the oregano and oil. Spoon the pesto over the chicken, then place on top of the tomato.

2. Gather up the edges of the foil and seal to make a parcel. Bake in the oven for 25–30 minutes until the potato is tender and the chicken is cooked through. Carefully open the parcel, remove the chicken and chop into four pieces.

3. Whiz the remaining contents of the parcel with the chicken in a food processor, or using a hand blender, until very finely chopped, adding a little milk if necessary.

perfect pesto

Homemade red pesto is super easy! Toast 100 g/3 1/2 oz pine nuts (or other type of nut or seed) in a dry nonstick frying pan. Remove from the pan and leave to cool. Heat 1 tablespoon extra virgin olive oil in the pan and fry 2 finely chopped garlic cloves for 1–2 minutes. Blitz the toasted nuts or seeds in a mini food processor until very finely chopped. Add 6 chopped sun-dried tomatoes in oil (drained) to the food processor, then add the garlic, 4 tablespoons of extra virgin olive oil and 100 ml/3 1/2 fl oz water. Blitz again until smooth, then stir in 50 g/1 3/4 oz finely grated Parmesan cheese. (For green pesto, replace the sun-dried tomatoes with 50 g/1 3/4 oz basil leaves.)

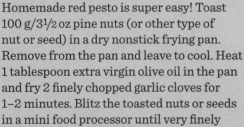

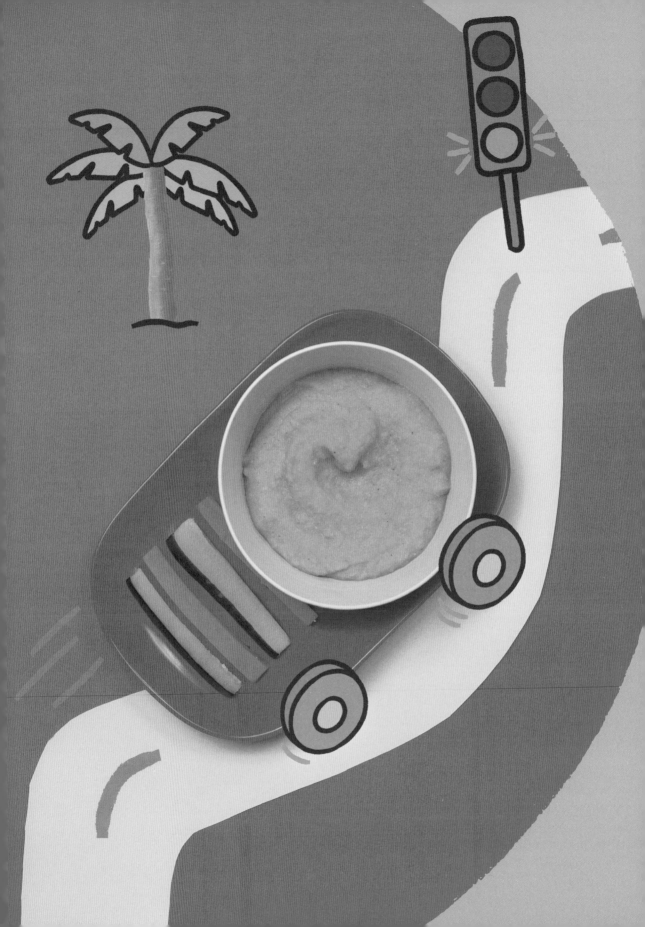

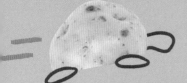

serves **2-3** | prep **10 mins** | cook **20 mins**

vroom-vroom veggie dhal

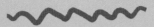

This delicious veggie dhal will take tiny taste buds
on a super-tasty adventure. Vroom, vroom!

what you need

50 g/1³/4 oz **dried split
red lentils**, rinsed

1 small **potato** (about 115 g/4 oz),
peeled and diced

1 **garlic clove**, peeled and quartered

1 small **carrot** (about 60 g/2¹/4 oz),
peeled and grated

3 tablespoons **baby's usual milk**,
plus extra if needed

¹/2 teaspoon **mild curry powder**

¹/4 teaspoon **ground turmeric**

1 teaspoon **unsalted butter**

what to do

1. Place the lentils, potato and garlic in a small
saucepan, cover with water and bring to the boil,
then reduce the heat and skim off any froth on
the surface. Add the carrot, part-cover with a lid
and simmer for 13–15 minutes until everything
is tender, then drain.

2. Return the lentils and vegetables to the pan. Add
the milk, curry powder, turmeric and butter and
stir until combined. Heat through for a couple of
minutes, crushing the potato and garlic with the
back of a fork.

3. Using the back of the fork, mash the lentil mixture
until almost smooth, adding a little extra milk if
necessary. Alternatively, puree in a food processor
or using a hand blender.

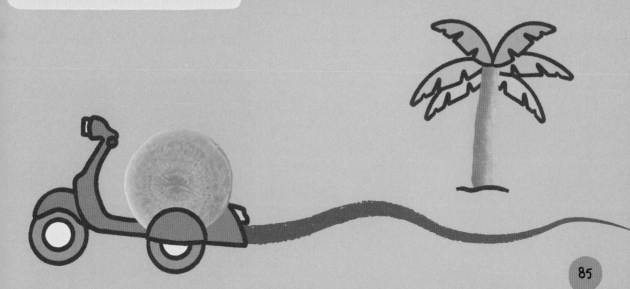

85

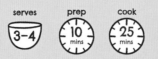

serves 3–4 **prep** 10 mins **cook** 25 mins

poppin' in-a-pot wonder!

Whip up this magic in-a-pot wonder with squishy lentils, fluffy cauliflower + a pop of pa-pa-paprika!

what you need

2 teaspoons **unsalted butter or olive oil**

75 g/2½ oz **cauliflower florets**, finely grated

50 g/1¾ oz **dried split red lentils**, rinsed

1 **garlic clove**, crushed

¼ teaspoon **ground cinnamon**

¼ teaspoon **mild smoked paprika**

250 ml/9 fl oz **passata** (sieved tomatoes)

20 g/¾ oz **couscous**

50 g/1¾ oz **frozen chopped spinach**

what to do

1. Heat 1 teaspoon of the butter or oil in a saucepan and add the cauliflower, lentils and garlic. Cook over a medium heat, stirring, for 1 minute or until combined.

2. Pour in 200 ml/7 fl oz water and bring to the boil, then turn the heat down. Add the spices and passata and cook, stirring often, for 15 minutes or until the lentils are tender.

3. Meanwhile, tip the couscous into a heatproof bowl and pour over enough just-boiled water to just cover the grains. Put a plate on top of the bowl and leave for 5 minutes or until the couscous is tender and the water has been absorbed. Fluff up the grains with a fork.

4. Add the spinach and the remaining butter or oil to the lentil mixture and cook for another 5 minutes or until heated through. Using a hand blender, blend the mixture to a coarse puree, adding a splash more hot water if needed, then stir in the couscous until combined.

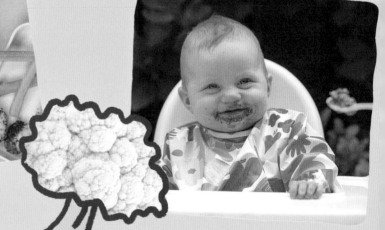

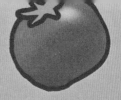

serves 2–3 | prep 10 mins | cook 30 mins

slurpy beef + veggie bol

Packed full of good stuff like cabbage + carrot, with broccoli florets to serve, this lip-smacking recipe will have your little one livin' on the veg!

what you need

2 teaspoons **olive oil**

100 g/3½ oz **minced beef**, finely chopped

1 small **onion**, finely chopped

1 **garlic clove**, crushed

30 g/1 oz **white cabbage**, finely grated

1 small **carrot** (about 50 g/1¾ oz), finely grated

½ teaspoon **dried oregano**

200 ml/7 fl oz **passata** (sieved tomatoes)

175 ml/6 fl oz **whole milk or milk of choice**

40 g/1½ oz **dried orzo pasta**

Broccoli florets, steamed until tender, to serve

what to do

1. Heat the oil in a saucepan over a medium heat, add the minced beef and cook, stirring to break up any clumps of meat, for 5 minutes or until browned. Using a slotted spoon, remove the mince and set aside on a plate.

2. Turn the heat down slightly and add the onion, garlic, cabbage, carrot and a splash of water if needed, then stir to combine. Cover the pan with a lid and cook for 5 minutes, stirring often.

3. Return the mince to the pan with the oregano, passata and milk and bring up to bubbling point. Turn the heat down to low, cover with a lid and simmer, stirring occasionally, for 20 minutes or until the vegetables are tender and the mince is cooked.

4. Meanwhile, cook the orzo in a saucepan of boiling water according to the packet instructions until tender. Drain, reserving the cooking water. Mash the pasta with the back of a fork while it's still in the sieve.

5. When the Bolognese is ready, mash with the back of a fork to a coarse puree, then stir in the mashed pasta and a splash of the reserved cooking water, if needed. Leave to cool slightly, then serve in bowls with steamed broccoli florets on the side as a finger food.

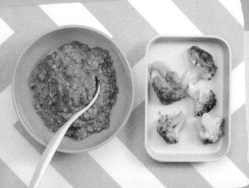

it's a mash-up!

Finely chopping the minced beef before cooking makes it easier to mash for baby. If you like, swap the mince, or half of it, with the same quantity of cooked green lentils.

87

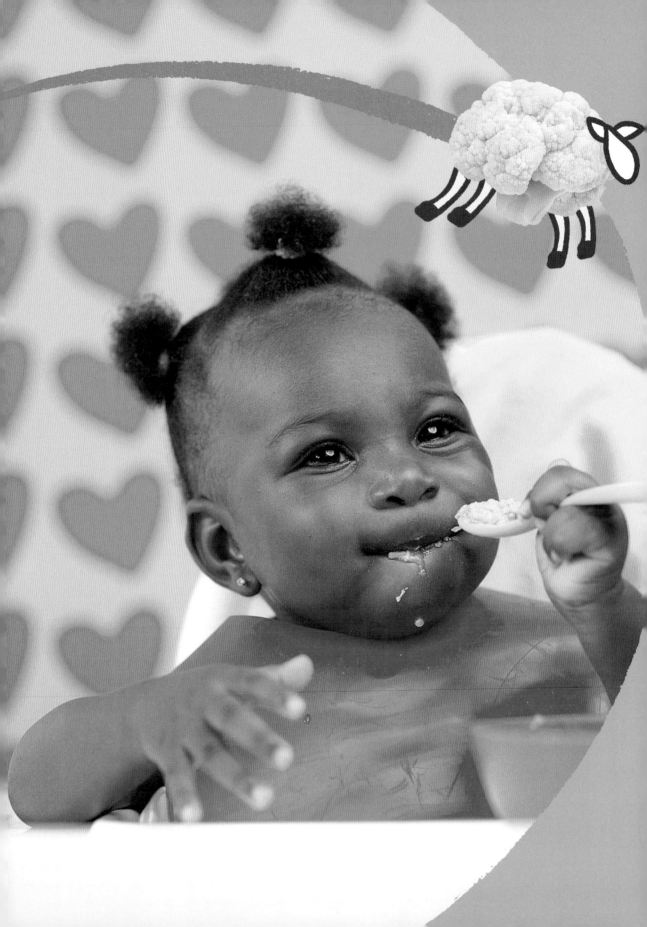

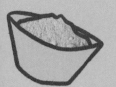

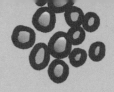

 serves **2**

 prep **10** mins

 cook **20** mins

my first chicken curry

This recipe is a great way to introduce your little one to new flavours like turmeric. Don't worry, though – there's only a hint of spice in this ch-ch-chicken curry!

what you need

2 teaspoons **olive oil**

1 skinless **chicken breast** (about 100 g/3½ oz)

30 g/1 oz **white basmati rice**, rinsed

30 g/1 oz **frozen peas**

30 g/1 oz **cauliflower florets**, finely grated

¼ teaspoon **mild curry powder**

¼ teaspoon **ground turmeric**

200 ml/7 fl oz **unsweetened coconut drinking milk or whole milk or milk of choice**

what to do

1. Heat the oil in a small saucepan over a medium heat. Add the chicken and cook, turning once, for 4 minutes or until starting to turn golden. Remove from the pan and set aside.

2. Add the rice to the pan with the peas, cauliflower and spices and mix until combined. Place the chicken breast on top of the rice mixture. Pour over 175 ml/6 fl oz of the coconut milk or milk and bring to the boil. Reduce the heat to low, cover with a lid and simmer for 12–15 minutes until the rice and chicken are cooked.

3. Remove the chicken, roughly chop, then place in a mini food processor with the remaining coconut milk or milk and process until very finely chopped.

4. Using a hand blender, mash the cooked rice and pea mixture in the pan to a coarse puree, adding more milk if needed and making sure the peas are broken down. Stir the chopped chicken into the rice mixture and serve.

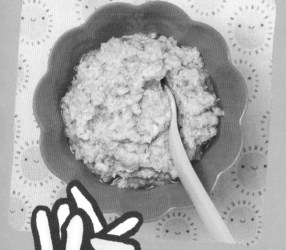

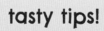 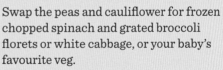

tasty tips!

Swap the peas and cauliflower for frozen chopped spinach and grated broccoli florets or white cabbage, or your baby's favourite veg.

Coconut drinking milk has a runnier consistency than canned coconut milk – make sure you buy one without added sugar.

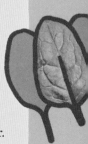

three ways with
pesto

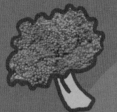

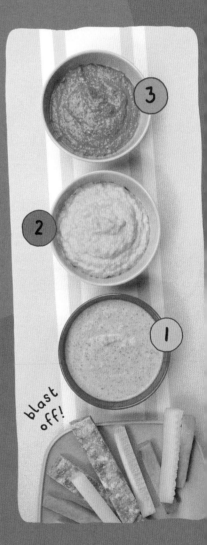

Ready? Steady? Let's get veggie! Using a yummy mix of veg, these traffic light dips are simple to make + absolutely deeelicious! What's more, they will keep in a container in the fridge for up to three days.

1 green for go

serves 3–4   **prep** 10 mins   **cook** 8 mins

what you need

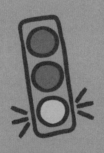

100 g/3½ oz **broccoli florets**

2 **garlic cloves**, peeled

30 g/1 oz **kale leaves** without stalks

1½ tablespoons **extra virgin olive oil**

20 g/¾ oz **Cheddar cheese**, finely grated

what to do

1. Steam the broccoli in a saucepan over a medium heat for 3 minutes or until starting to soften. Add the garlic and kale and steam for another 5 minutes or until tender. Reserve the cooking water.

2. Put the broccoli, garlic and kale in a mini food processor with the oil and 3–4 tablespoons of the reserved cooking water and blend until smooth, adding more cooking water if needed to make a pesto consistency. Stir in the cheese until combined, adding a splash more oil or cooking water if needed.

blast off!

amazing orange

serves 3–4 | prep 10 mins | cook 30 mins

what you need

3 **carrots** (about 200 g/7 oz), peeled and quartered lengthways

1 1/2 tablespoons **extra virgin olive oil**, plus extra for cooking the carrots

2 **garlic cloves**, unpeeled

50 g/1 3/4 oz **blanched almonds**

10 g/1/4 oz **Cheddar cheese**, finely grated

what to do

1. Preheat the oven to 180°C/350°F/Gas Mark 4. Toss the carrots in a little oil, then place in a baking dish with the garlic and roast for 30 minutes or until soft.

2. Meanwhile, toast the almonds for 15–20 minutes on a baking sheet in the bottom of the oven, turning once, until starting to turn golden. Leave to cool.

3. Finely grind the almonds in a mini food processor. Squeeze the garlic cloves out of their skins and roughly chop the carrots. Add both to the food processor. Add the oil and 4 tablespoons of water, then blend until smooth, adding more water if necessary to make a pesto consistency. Stir in the cheese until combined, adding a splash more oil or water if needed.

ruby red

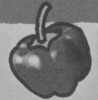

serves 3–4 | prep 10 mins | cook 20 mins

what you need

2 large **red peppers**, halved, deseeded and each half cut into 4 strips, or **roasted peppers** in oil from a jar, drained

1 1/2 tablespoons **extra virgin olive oil**, plus extra for cooking the peppers

2 **garlic cloves**, unpeeled

50 g/1 3/4 oz **cashew nuts**

2 teaspoons **tomato puree**

10 g/1/4 oz **Cheddar cheese**, finely grated

what to do

1. Preheat the oven to 180°C/350°F/Gas Mark 4. Toss the peppers in a little oil, place in a baking dish with the garlic and roast for 20 minutes or until soft. Transfer to a bowl, cover with clingfilm and leave to stand until cool enough to handle. If using jarred peppers you can skip this step.

2. Meanwhile, toast the cashews for 15–20 minutes on a baking sheet in the oven, turning once, until starting to go golden. Leave to cool, then finely grind in a mini food processor.

3. Squeeze the garlic cloves out of their skins and peel the skins off the peppers. Add both to the food processor. Add the tomato puree, oil and 2 tablespoons of water, then blend until smooth, adding more water if necessary to make a pesto consistency. Stir in the cheese until combined, adding a splash more oil or water if needed.

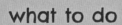

serves **3–4** | prep **10 mins** | cook **20 mins**

very nice fish + rice

Bursting with exciting tastes, including green beans + tangy tomatoes, this recipe is packed full of vitamin C, which helps support little immune systems.

what you need

40 g/1½ oz **white basmati rice**, rinsed

4 **green beans**, trimmed and chopped

2 **broccoli florets**, chopped

2 teaspoons **olive oil**

125 g/4½ oz skinless, boneless **white fish fillet**, such as haddock

200 ml/7 fl oz **passata** (sieved tomatoes)

½ teaspoon **dried oregano**

what to do

1. Put the rice in a saucepan and pour in enough cold water to cover by 2 cm/¾ inch. Bring to the boil, add the beans and broccoli, then turn the heat down to low, cover and simmer for 12–15 minutes until tender.

2. Meanwhile, heat the oil in a nonstick frying pan over a medium heat and cook the fish for 5 minutes, turning once, until cooked through. Remove the fish with a spatula and flake into small pieces, taking care to remove any bones.

3. Drain the rice and vegetables, saving 4 tablespoons of the cooking water. Return the rice and vegetables to the pan with the flaked fish, passata and oregano. Cook over a low heat, stirring frequently, for 5 minutes or until warmed through.

4. Using the back of a fork, mash the fish mixture until almost smooth, adding a little reserved cooking water if necessary. Alternatively, puree in a food processor or using a hand blender.

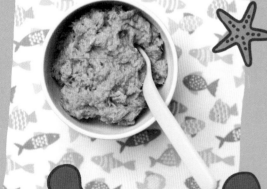

super-shaker

Pop some uncooked rice in a clean plastic bottle and secure the lid. While you're rustling up this tasty dish, give the shaker to your baby to make some music for you to cook along to. Don't forget to dance! Lentils, crisped rice and water are good shaker-fillers, too.

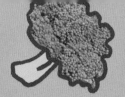

serves **2** | prep **10** mins | cook **30** mins

scrummy lemon-y salmon + beans

Make mealtimes go swimmingly with this juicy salmon. It is super soft for your little one's gums + the lemon gives the dish a tasty twist!

what you need

125 g/4^{1}/$_{2}$ oz skinless, boneless **salmon fillet**

1 **unwaxed lemon**, zest grated

10 g/^{1}/$_{4}$ oz **unsalted butter**, cubed

1 small **potato** (about 125 g/ 4^{1}/$_{2}$ oz), peeled and cut into 1 cm/^{1}/$_{2}$ inch pieces

4 **green beans**, trimmed and sliced

1 **baby leek**, finely chopped

3 small **broccoli florets**

2 tablespoons **baby's usual milk**, plus extra if needed

Freshly ground **black pepper**

what to do

1. Preheat the oven to 180°C/350°F/Gas Mark 4. Place a sheet of aluminium foil large enough to wrap the salmon in a baking dish. Add the salmon, then sprinkle over the lemon zest and dot with the butter. Place 2 lemon slices on top and season with a little pepper. Gather up the edges of the foil and seal to make a parcel. Bake in the oven for 15–20 minutes until the salmon is cooked through.

2. Meanwhile, put the potato in a saucepan and pour in enough cold water to cover. Part-cover the pan with the lid, bring to the boil over a medium heat and cook for 5 minutes. Add the beans, leek and broccoli and cook for another 5 minutes or until the vegetables are tender. Drain, then return the vegetables to the pan with the milk and a squeeze of lemon juice and heat through briefly.

3. Open the parcel, place the salmon on a plate and flake it into small pieces, adding some of the buttery juices from the parcel. Stir the salmon and juices into the potato mixture. Whiz with a hand blender to a fine mash texture, adding a splash more milk if needed.

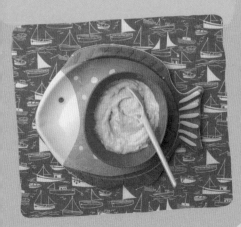

our friends say...

'When I was breastfeeding, I ate lots of different spices so that my little one got used to strong tastes in her milk feeds. It seemed to work – she's showing signs of becoming a really adventurous eater!'

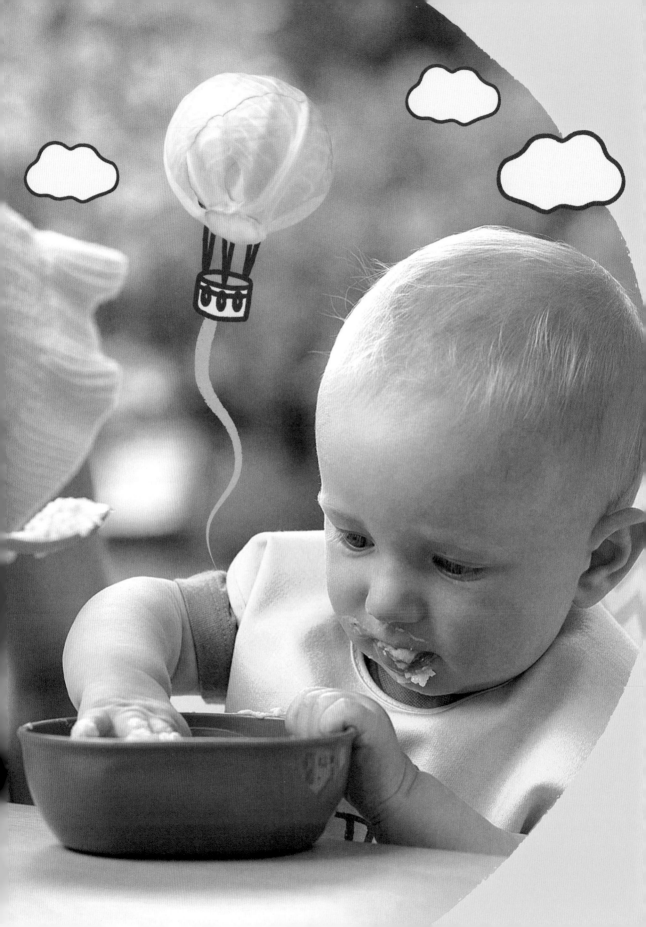

serves 2

 prep 10 mins

 cook 10 mins

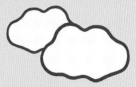

dreamy creamy bean mash

This simple mashed recipe combines beans + greens
for a dinner of dreams!

what you need

4 good-sized **broccoli florets**
(about 85 g/3 oz)

1 **garlic clove**, peeled

2 **spring onions**, roughly chopped

60 g/2¼ oz **white cabbage**, sliced

150 g/5½ oz drained **canned
cannellini beans** in water, rinsed

8 tablespoons **whole milk or milk
of choice**, plus extra if needed

20 g/¾ oz **mature Cheddar cheese**
(or dairy-free alternative), grated

Bread, cut into fingers, to serve

what to do

1. Steam the broccoli, garlic and spring onions
   in a saucepan over a medium heat for 3 minutes,
   then add the cabbage and steam for another
   2–3 minutes until the vegetables are tender.

2. Meanwhile, put the beans and 6 tablespoons of the
   milk into a small saucepan and warm through for
   5 minutes or until the beans have softened. Mash
   the beans with the back of a fork or blend to a
   coarse puree with a hand blender.

3. When the vegetables and garlic are cooked, blend
   them (setting aside 2 broccoli florets to serve)
   with the remaining milk. Stir the vegetable puree
   into the beans with the cheese. Warm through
   gently until the cheese melts, adding a splash more
   milk if it is too thick. Serve the creamy bean mash
   with the reserved cooked broccoli florets and
   bread on the side as finger food.

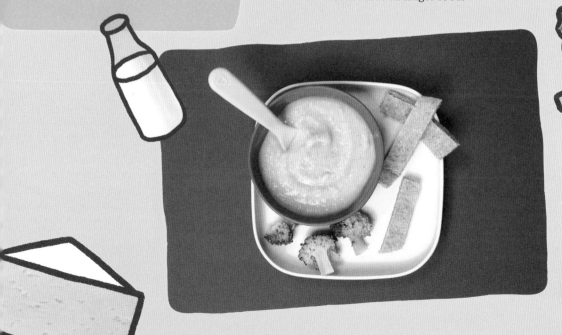

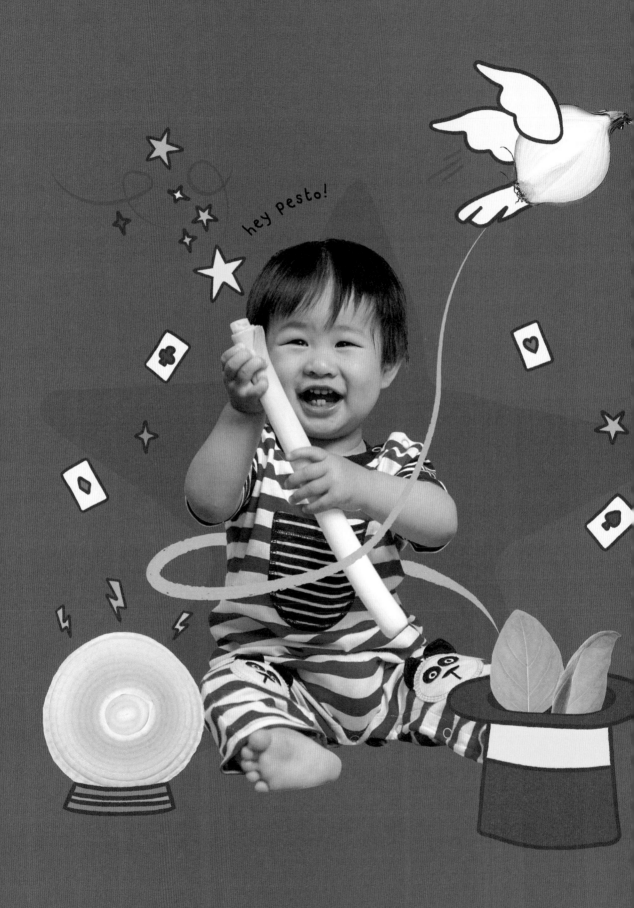

hey pesto!

time
to
chew

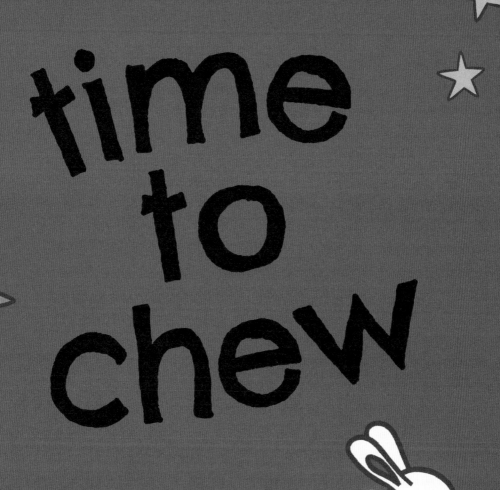

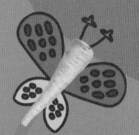

from 10 months

At 10 months old, little ones often have a few of their first tiny teeth + new chunkier textures can give those gnashers something to chew on. If your little one isn't showing any signs of teeth peeping through yet, don't worry. They're brilliant at chewing soft chunks with just their gums! Offering a wide variety of foods is still important for providing a range of nutrients as well as for exciting tiny taste buds. The recipes in this chapter have lots of punchy tastes, perfect for encouraging little ones to be more adventurous with food.

what to give

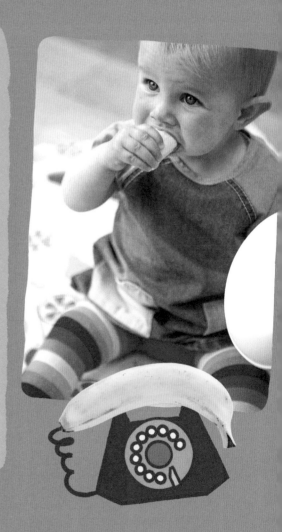

As little explorers become more mobile – some will be crawling, climbing and cruising – as well as growing super fast, their energy requirements increase. Offer a variety of foods in three meals a day, including the following food groups (see page 16 for examples):

☺ Carbohydrate foods at each meal

☺ 1–2 veggies or fruits at each meal

☺ A protein food at 2–3 meals a day

☺ 3 dairy foods (or alternatives) a day

☺ Plus sources of healthy fats

Let little ones eat according to their appetite (see page 17 for signs they've had enough) and offer seconds if they're still hungry.

Don't forget, milk is still an important source of nutrition so offer 400 ml/14 fl oz of their usual milk each day.

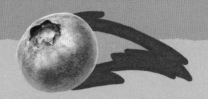

tips on texture

By now, most little ones will be able to munch food with an up and down movement of the jaw. They can use their tongues to move soft pieces of food to the side of their mouth for chewing in the place where their munchy molars will be in the future.

From 10 months, little ones can also pick up small, soft foods like halved blueberries or raspberries, between their thumbs and forefingers using a pincer grip, and are getting more accurate with taking charge to feed themselves.

Bear in mind that they still can't manage hard lumps and chunks like whole nuts, hard pieces in thin liquid, such as cereal in milk, or fibrous, crumbly or brittle foods.

Little ones can now handle small, soft chunks that are in a thick puree, as long as the puree is kept moist, to minimize the risk of choking. Go for lumps about the size of a pea that squish and mush easily under the back of a fork. You'll still need to mash or finely shred any meat or fish but other ingredients can be finely chopped and well cooked until soft, even whole peas.

Keep offering finger foods with each meal or even try finger food meals to help little ones develop those all-important self-feeding skills. Finger food meals are a great option for adventurous eaters if you make sure the texture is still soft and easily mushable between your thumb and finger. Our Grab + Go Cheesy Eggy Fingers, Cheeky Chicken Croquettes and Oh-fish-ially Tasty Fish Fingers (see pages 116, 122 and 129) are great ideas for finger food meals. Go for either finger-shaped foods or small chunks of super-soft pieces, like soft fruit, about the size of a pea.

tingling taste buds

Strong tastes aren't scary! Little ones might need a few tries before they accept a new food, especially if it's a punchy taste, but keep going. Try our Just-for-me VIPea Salmon Risotto for a taste twist (see page 121)!

how much?

You baby will probably be having three meals a day by now plus 400 ml/14 fl oz of their usual milk but it's normal for their appetite to vary. Continue to respond to your little one's appetite but take a peek at our 'handy' guide to portion sizes for each meal!

☺ Meat, fish or other protein foods – a baby's palm-sized amount

☺ Carbohydrate foods like pasta, potato or rice – a baby's fist-sized amount

☺ Fruit and veg – 1–2 baby handfuls

Bear in mind that not only do little ones' appetites vary from one day to the next, depending upon growth spurts, activity levels, teething and whether they are feeling a bit under the weather, but also every baby is different. Some little ones eat a lot, some very little and that's completely normal. As long as your baby is growing well, is full of beans and your health visitor or doctor is happy then you're doing fine.

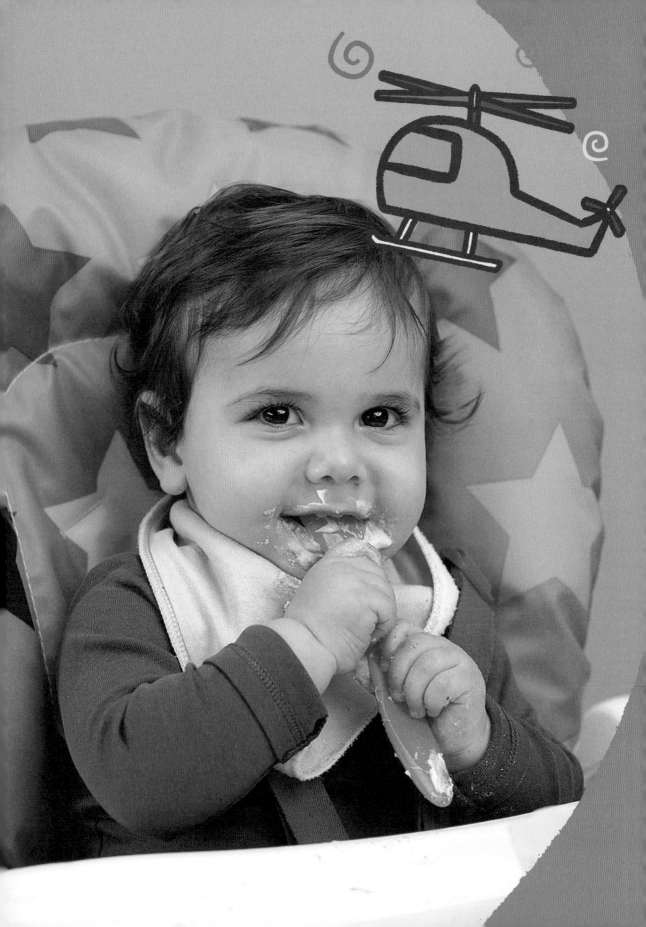

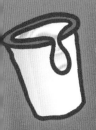

serves **2-3**   prep **10 mins** + soaking   cook **no cook**

twirly whirly yogurt pots

Try these twirly whirly pots of yumminess!
The dates + cashews make a thick, gooey,
caramel-y sauce. Yummmmmm!

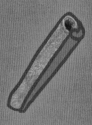

what you need

40 g/1½ oz **soft pitted dates**

30 g/1 oz **cashew nuts**

1–2 tablespoons **whole milk or milk of choice**, plus extra if needed

Large pinch of **ground cinnamon**

Natural Greek yogurt

Lightly toasted **muffin or potato cakes**, cut into fingers, to serve

what to do

1. Put the dates and cashews in a heatproof bowl and pour over 2 tablespoons just-boiled water. Cover and leave to soak overnight, or for at least 2 hours.

2. Just before serving, put the dates, cashews and the soaking water in a mini food processor or blender. Add the milk and cinnamon and blend until smooth, adding a splash more milk if needed to give a thick puree consistency.

3. For each serving, spoon some yogurt into a small breakfast bowl and top with the date mixture. Serve with fingers of lightly toasted muffin or potato cake.

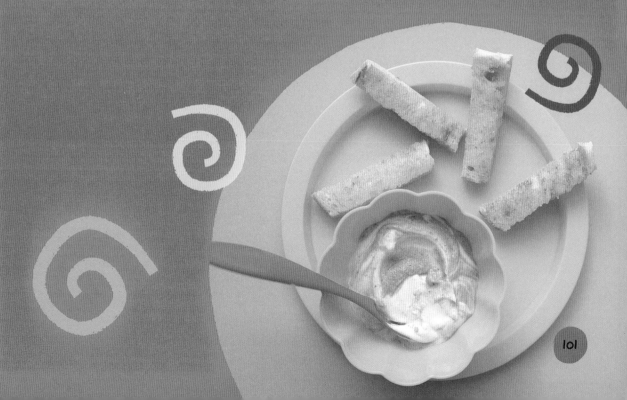

three ways with
oats

A store-cupboard superhero, oats are great for filling up little tums! Try these three easy ways to wake up your little one's taste buds.

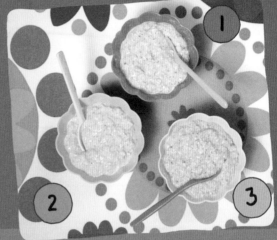

1

coconut + pear overnight oats

serves **2**

prep **10 mins**
+ overnight soaking

cook **no cook**

what you need

30 g/1 oz **rolled oats**

75 ml/2½ fl oz unsweetened **coconut drinking milk**

1 teaspoon **ground mixed seeds** (optional)

2 tablespoons **coconut yogurt or yogurt of choice**

Large pinch of **ground cinnamon**

1 ripe and juicy **pear**, peeled

what to do

1. Tip the oats into a bowl and pour over the milk, then stir until combined. Cover with clingfilm and place in the fridge overnight.

2. The next morning, stir the seeds into the oats (if using) and mix in the yogurt and cinnamon. Mash the oats slightly with the back of the spoon for a smoother consistency, if preferred.

3. Finely grate the pear, mashing the fruit slightly with the back of a fork. Stir the pear into the creamy oats, adding more milk to loosen the oats if needed.

t-OAT-ally tasty!

For a warm oat brekkie, soak the oats in half the milk overnight, then heat the remaining milk until hot and stir it into the breakfast with the grated pear just before serving.

strawberries + cream overnight oats

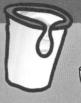

serves **2**

prep **10 mins** + overnight soaking

cook **no cook**

what you need

30 g/1 oz **rolled oats**

75 ml/2¹/₂ fl oz **whole milk or milk of choice**

1 teaspoon **ground mixed seeds** (optional)

2 tablespoons **natural Greek yogurt**

5 ripe **strawberries**, about 75 g/2¹/₂ oz, hulled

¹/₄ teaspoon **vanilla extract** (optional)

what to do

1. Tip the oats into a bowl and pour over the milk, then stir until combined. Cover with clingfilm and place in the fridge overnight.

2. The next morning, stir the seeds into the oats (if using) and mix in the yogurt. Mash the oats slightly with the back of the spoon for a smoother consistency, if preferred.

3. Using a food processor or blender, blend the strawberries with the vanilla (if using) and stir into the creamy oats, adding more milk to loosen the oats as required.

nectarine + carrot overnight oats

serves **2**

prep **10 mins** + overnight soaking

cook **no cook**

what you need

30 g/1 oz **rolled oats**

100 ml/3¹/₂ fl oz **whole milk or milk of choice**

1 small **cooked carrot** (about 50 g/1³/₄ oz), roughly chopped

1 ripe juicy **nectarine**, halved, stoned and roughly sliced

Large pinch of **ground nutmeg**

1 teaspoon **ground mixed seeds** (optional)

what to do

1. Tip the oats into a bowl, pour over the milk and stir until combined.

2. Place the cooked carrot and nectarine in a food processor or blender and blend until smooth. Stir the puree, nutmeg and ground seeds (if using) into the oats. Cover with clingfilm and place in the fridge overnight.

3. The next morning, mash the oats slightly with the back of the spoon for a smoother consistency, if preferred, adding a splash more milk to loosen the oats if needed.

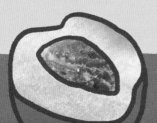

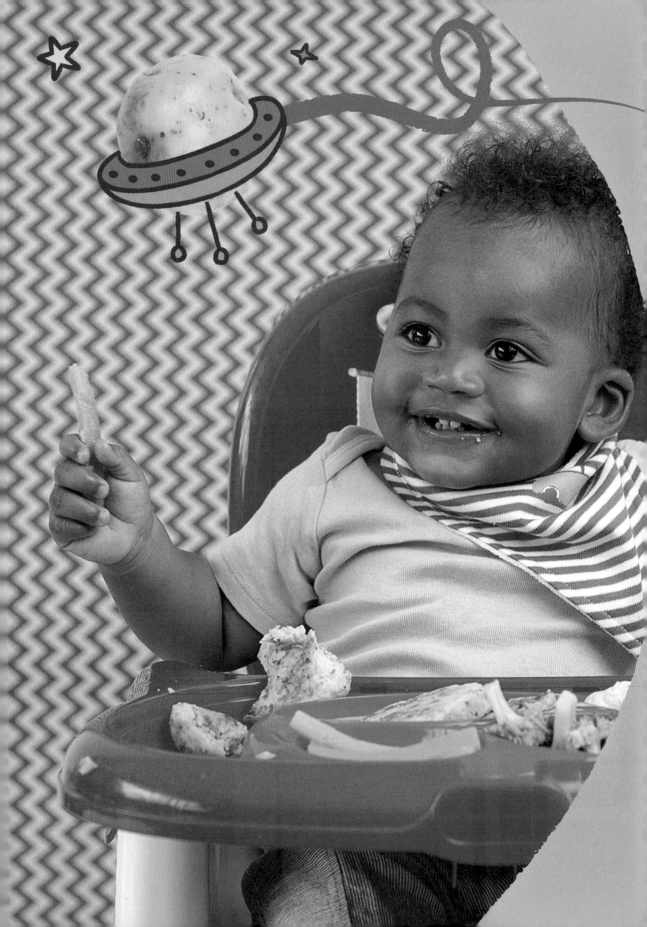

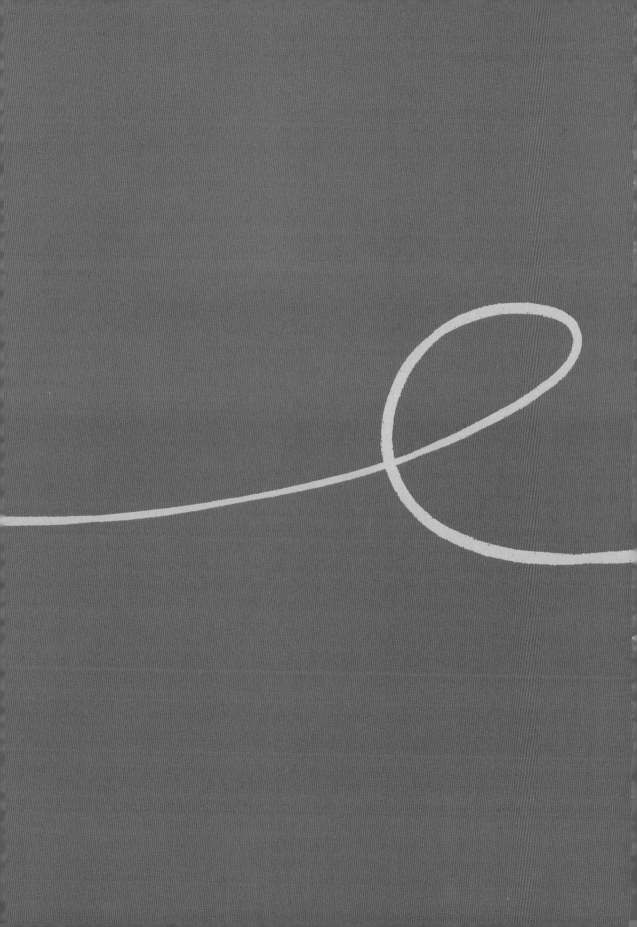

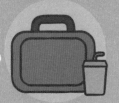 lunch	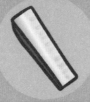 snack	dinner	before bed
...te-me-up prawn + ...ato orzo (see page 183) with steamed green veg	quarter of a bagel with cheese spread + plum fingers	feelin' fine falafel (see page 176) with sweet potatoes + your choice of sauce	milk
...eesy corn triangles ...e page 160) with hummus + steamed carrot sticks	sweet potato + bean dip (see page 119) + cucumber sticks	bangin' BBQ chicken with minty potato salad (see page 171) + steamed green beans	milk
super-duper ...hick-chick pasta ...page 163) + broccoli florets	half a crumpet with cheese spread + quartered grapes	mighty mackerel salad (see page 167)	milk
sizzle-sizzle ...mato-y scramble ...ee page 157) with flatbread + cucumber sticks	leftover new potatoes (reserved from last night's salad) with hard-boiled egg wedges	little fishy in a dishy (see page 182) with couscous + chopped fruit with yogurt	milk
...uscous with tuna ...o mash + quartered grapes	mackerel pâté with fine-milled oatcakes + cucumber sticks	quick + easy cheesy lasagne (see page 191) with steamed green veg	milk
goin' goin' ...one! green pasta ...page 164) with a spoonful of ...ed lentils + strawberry slices	fruit bread with spread + melon fingers	squish-squish dinky dumplings (see page 187) + broccoli florets	milk
...asted chicken strips ...ith roasted new potatoes, parsnips + carrots	best-of-the-bunch banana muffins (see page 200) + raspberries	rainbow veg + tofu kebabs (see page 175) with brown rice + blueberries + yogurt	milk

smooooth

crrrunch

	wakey wakey!	**breakfast**	**snack**	
day 1	milk	**porridge** with mashed banana + cinnamon	**greek yogurt** with drained canned peaches in juice (chopped or mashed)	pl... tor...
day 2	milk	**slice of wholemeal toast** with peanut butter + quartered grapes	**cottage cheese** with shop-bought breadsticks + melon fingers	ch... (se...
day 3	milk	**apple + cinnamon pancakes** (see page 69) with Greek yogurt	**cucumber sticks** + pitta fingers with hummus	... (se...
day 4	milk	**nectarine + carrot overnight oats** (see page 103)	**half an English muffin** with peanut butter + grated apple	t... (...
day 5	milk	**spinach, oat + cheese pancakes** (see page 68) with hummus	**malt loaf** with spread + chopped strawberries	c... +...
day 6	milk	**lovely hearts brekkie bread rolls** (see page 151) with scrambled egg + quartered cherry tomatoes	**pitta fingers** with Minty Cucumber + Cream Cheese Dip (see page 118)	... (se... tin...
day 7	milk	**ready-in-a-flash brekkie hash** (see page 148) with hard-boiled eggs + toast fingers	**half a crumpet** with grated cheese	ro...

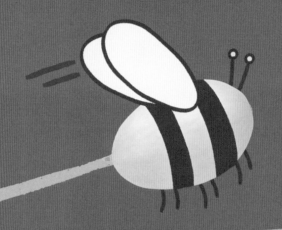

open me to find
your pull-out weaning
**meal planner
+ wall chart**
for little ones aged
12 months+!

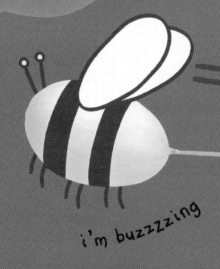

ng wall chart

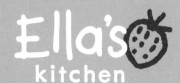**Ella's kitchen**

n with all your favourite foodie memories

te fruits

shine on!

months,
ating...

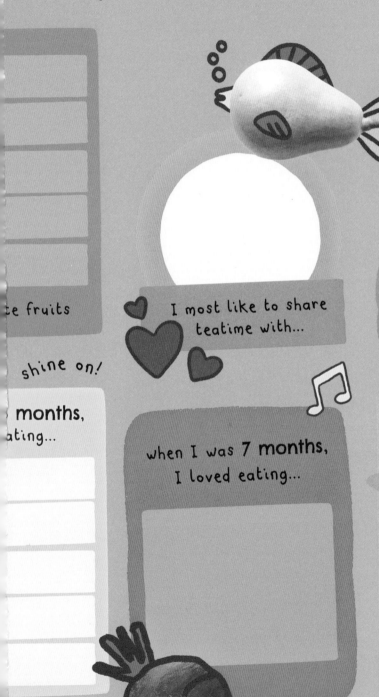

I most like to share
teatime with...

when I was **7 months,**
I loved eating...

when I was **10 months,**
I loved eating...

winnerrr
winner

now I'm **one year** old,
I love eating...

1

2

3

4

5

zing.

this wall chart belongs to...

my weani

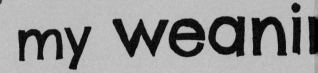

stick up this wall chart and fill it

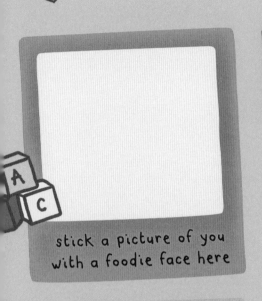

stick a picture of you
with a foodie face here

I did some scooping with
my very own spoon on...

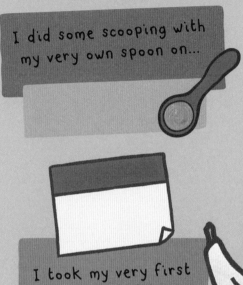

I took my very first
yummy mouthful on...

1
2
3
4
5

my favouri

my very first puree was...

my favourite veggies

yum!

my first chompy tooth
popped through today

when I was
I loved e

1
2
3
4
5

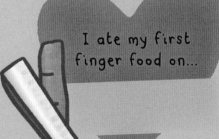

I ate my first
finger food on...

makes 10

prep 10 mins

cook 20 mins

spud-tastic veggie fritters

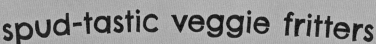

Serve these yummy fritters to all your best spuddies! They are so versatile + simple – just leftover veg + mashed potato. Spudtacular!

what you need

375 g/13 oz **leftover mash** or 450 g/1 lb **potatoes**, peeled, cooked and mashed with 10 g/¼ oz **unsalted butter**

5 **spring onions**, very finely chopped

50 g/1¾ oz cooked vegetables, such as **cabbage, broccoli, cauliflower or carrot**, very finely chopped or mashed

40 g/1½ oz **plain flour**, plus extra for dusting

50 g/1¾ oz **mature Cheddar cheese**, grated

1 teaspoon **English mustard**

1 small **egg**, lightly beaten

Olive oil, for frying

what to do

1. Put the cold mash in a mixing bowl and stir in the spring onions, cooked vegetables, flour, cheese, mustard and egg, then mix well until combined.

2. Using well-floured hands, take small handfuls of the mash mixture and shape into cakes about 1 cm/½ inch thick and 7 cm/2¾ inches in diameter – the mixture makes about 10 in total.

3. Pour enough oil into a large nonstick frying pan to cover the base and heat over a medium heat. Preheat the oven to the lowest setting to keep the cooked fritters warm while you fry them in batches. Cook the fritters for 7–8 minutes, turning once or twice, until light golden and crisp on the outside and hot in the middle. Turn the heat down slightly if they start to get too dark.

4. Place the cooked fritters on a kitchen paper-lined plate to drain and keep warm in the oven while you cook the second batch. Cut into halves or quarters and offer as finger food or mash them up and serve with your baby's favourite accompaniments.

suuuper swaps!

Mix + match your baby's fave foods + dips to serve with the veggie fritters:

☺ Scrambled, poached or boiled eggs

☺ Hummus or dip

☺ Low-sugar, low-salt baked beans, mashed

☺ Pureed cooked/roasted tomatoes

☺ Steamed vegetable sticks

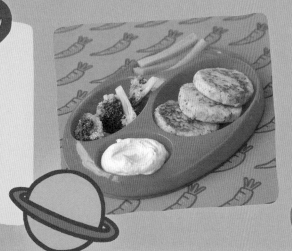

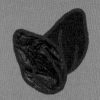

makes
6

prep
10 mins
+ chilling

cook
20 mins

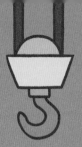

pick-up porridge bars

Perfect whether you are at home or on the go, these squiiiishy porridge bars will keep your little one go, go, going!

what you need

40 g/1½ oz **porridge oats**

175 ml/6 fl oz **whole milk or milk of choice**

15 g/½ oz **raisins or other dried fruit**, very finely chopped

½ teaspoon **ground cinnamon**

1 teaspoon **ground mixed seeds**

10 g/¼ oz **unsalted butter**

what to do

1) Line a small baking sheet with baking parchment. Place the oats and milk in a small saucepan and bring to the boil, then reduce the heat and simmer, stirring frequently, for 8 minutes or until the oats are very soft and mushy – it should be a thick porridge consistency.

2) Transfer to a bowl and stir in the raisins, cinnamon and seeds, then spread out the porridge on the prepared baking sheet in an even layer about 1 cm/½ inch thick. Cover and chill for 30 minutes or until set.

3) Cut the porridge into 6 fingers, each about 7 cm/ 2¾ inches long by 2.5 cm/1 inch wide.

4) Melt the butter in a large, nonstick frying pan and cook the fingers for 3 minutes on each side or until golden. Leave to cool slightly before serving.

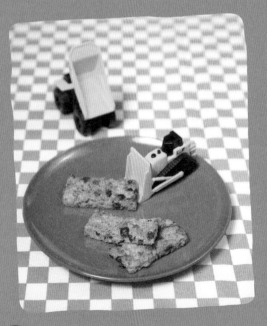

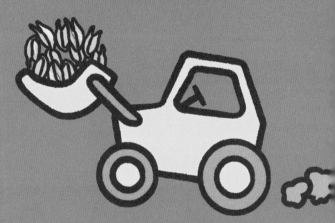

serves **2–3** | prep **5 mins** | cook **5 mins**

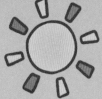

sunny-side-up couscous bowl

Tick tock it's couscous o'clock! Make your little one's day with this sunny side up brekkie using turmeric + cheese.

what you need

250 ml/9 fl oz no- or low-salt **vegetable stock or water**

125 ml/4 fl oz **whole milk or milk of choice**

50 g/1¾ oz **frozen chopped spinach**

¼ teaspoon **ground turmeric**

75 g/2½ oz **couscous**

30 g/1 oz **Cheddar cheese**, finely grated

2 **hard-boiled eggs**, shelled and cut into quarters

what to do

1. Pour the stock or water into a small saucepan with the milk, spinach and turmeric. Stir well and warm over a medium–low heat.

2. When the liquid starts to bubble, stir in the couscous and turn the heat to low. Cook, stirring with a wooden spoon, for 3–4 minutes until soft.

3. Stir in the cheese and heat until melted. Mash with the back of a fork to break down the couscous, adding extra water or milk if needed. Serve in bowls with the hard-boiled eggs on the side as finger food.

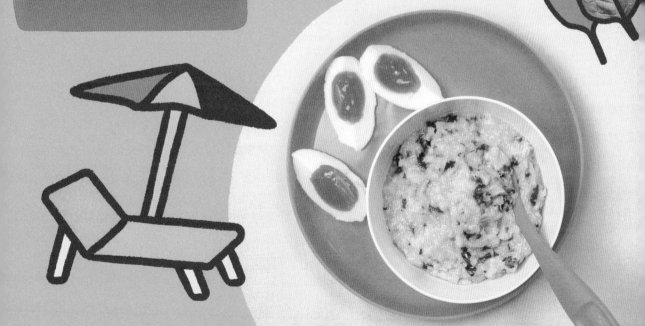

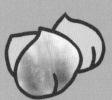

dip-dip-dip peanut hummus

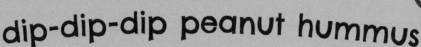

Creamy + crunchy, this dip is so yummy your little ones won't be able to stop themselves from dip-dip-dipping!

what you need

125 g/4½ oz drained **canned chickpeas** in water, plus 2 tablespoons water from the can

2 tablespoons **lemon juice**

1 tablespoon **light tahini**

1 tablespoon no-salt, no-sugar smooth **peanut butter or extra tahini**

1 small **garlic clove**, crushed

1 tablespoon **olive oil**

what to do

1. Place the chickpeas, lemon juice, tahini, peanut butter (if using), garlic and oil in a mini food processor or blender. Pour in the chickpea water or use regular water and blend until smooth and creamy.

2. Spoon some of the hummus into a small bowl and serve to your baby with your choice of dunkers for dipping in.

to serve

Choose from the following dunkers:

Toast, buttered and cut into fingers

Warm pitta bread or flatbread, cut into fingers

Potato cakes or muffins, cut into fingers

Hard-boiled egg, shelled and cut into quarters

Wedges of **avocado**

Steamed **vegetable fingers**

Wedges of **melon or soft fruit**

deeeliciously dippable!

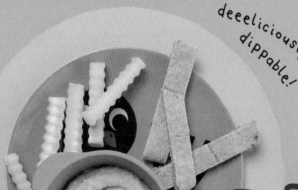

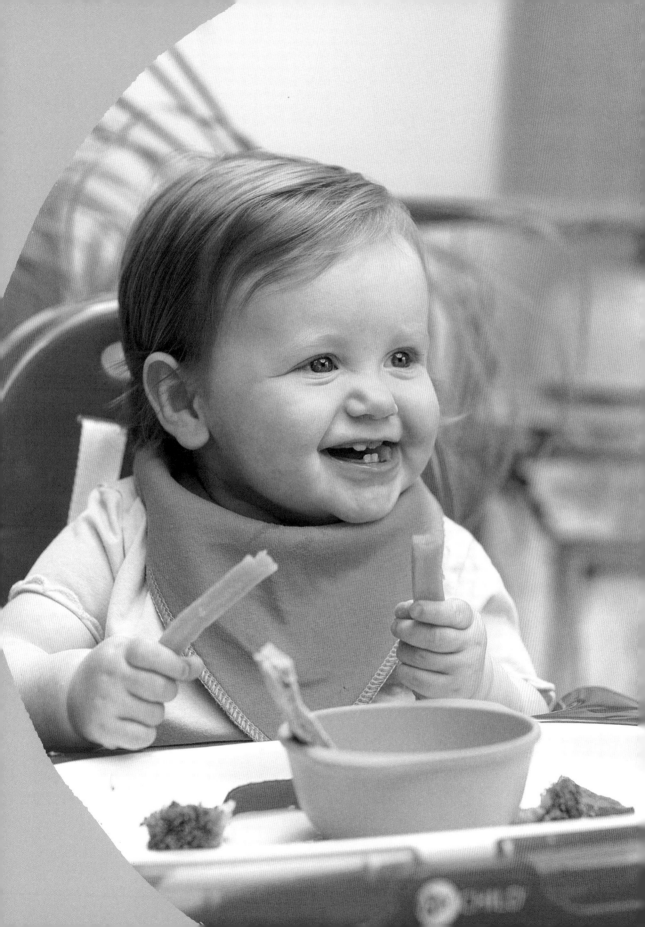

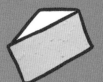

a-MAIZE-ing sweetcorn crumpets

Toot, toot! Sound the trumpets for these
unbeatable brekkie crumpets!

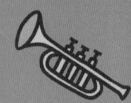

what you need

1 **egg**

30 g/1 oz drained no-salt, no-sugar
canned sweetcorn

2 tablespoons **whole milk or milk
of choice**

10 g/1/4 oz **Parmesan cheese,**
finely grated

2 **crumpets**

10 g/1/4 oz **unsalted butter**

Freshly ground **black pepper**

Banana fingers, to serve

what to do

1) Place the egg, sweetcorn and milk in a food
processor or blender and blend until smooth.
Stir in the Parmesan and season with pepper.
Pour the mixture into a shallow bowl.

2) Place the crumpets, top-side down, in the egg
mixture, then turn over to coat the other side.
Spoon any leftover egg mixture into the holes
in the crumpets and leave to soak briefly.

3) Melt the butter in a small nonstick frying pan
over a medium–low heat. When hot, place the
crumpets, bottom-side down, in the pan and
cook for 2–3 minutes. Turn the crumpets over
and cook for another 2–3 minutes until the
eggy corn coating turns golden and sets.

4) Leave to cool slightly, then slice and serve with
fingers of banana.

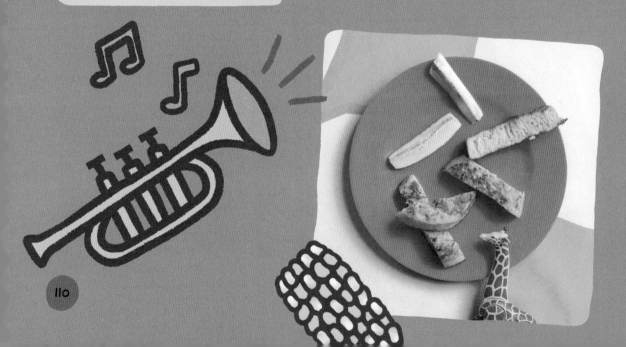

serves 2
 prep 5 mins
 cook 15 mins

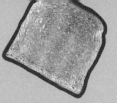

cheeky beans + eggs

This easy beany eggy brekkie is sure to fill up your cheeky chops!

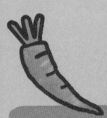

what you need

2 **eggs**

1 **carrot** (about 75 g/2½ oz), peeled and chopped

100 g/3½ oz drained **canned haricot beans** in water, rinsed

2 tablespoons **tomato puree**

10 g/¼ oz **unsalted butter**

4 tablespoons **whole milk or baby's usual milk**, plus extra if needed

Toasted bread, buttered and cut into fingers, to serve

what to do

1. Put the eggs and carrot in a small saucepan and pour over just-boiled water to cover. Return the water to the boil and cook over a medium heat for 10 minutes.

2. Meanwhile, place the beans, tomato puree and butter in a separate small saucepan and cook gently, stirring frequently, for 5 minutes or until softened.

3. Drain and refresh the eggs under cold running water and peel off the shells. Put the eggs and carrot in a bowl and mash with the back of a fork.

4. Add the mashed eggs and carrot and the milk to the pan with the bean mixture, stir and heat through. Mash to a coarse puree, adding a little extra milk if necessary. Serve with toast fingers.

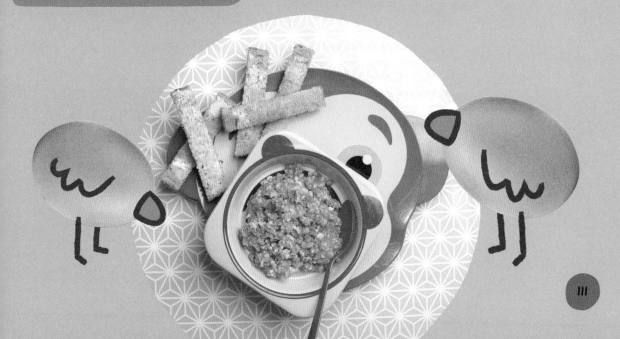

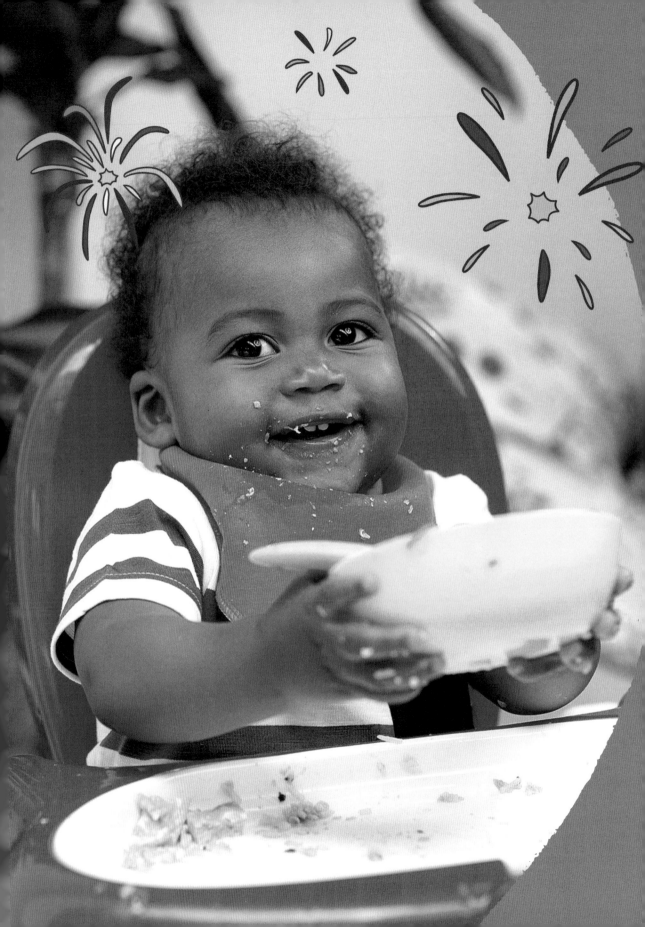

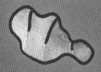

serves 2-3   prep 10 mins   cook 15 mins

un-bowl-ievable veggie rice bowl

This veggie rice bowl is packed full of exciting tastes for little mouths. Swap out the veg for whatever you have to hand. It's so easy to make, it's un-bowl-ievable!

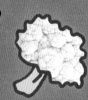

what you need

2 teaspoons **olive oil**

2 **spring onions**, finely chopped

1 heaped teaspoon grated **fresh root ginger**

85 g/3 oz **cauliflower florets**, finely grated

75 g/2¹/2 oz **white basmati rice**, rinsed

100 g/3¹/2 oz drained no-salt, no-sugar **canned sweetcorn**

50 g/1³/4 oz **frozen chopped spinach**

¹/2 teaspoon **Chinese 5-spice**

¹/2 teaspoon reduced-salt **soy sauce**

Omelette, cut into strips, to serve

what to do

1. Heat the oil in a saucepan over a medium heat, add the spring onions and cook, stirring, for 2 minutes or until softened. Add the ginger, cauliflower and rice and stir well until combined.

2. Pour 325 ml/11 fl oz water into the pan and bring to the boil. When the water starts to bubble, turn the heat down to low, cover with a lid and simmer for 10 minutes or until the rice is tender – it should still be quite watery.

3. Meanwhile, put the sweetcorn and 2 tablespoons of water in a bowl and blend with a hand blender.

4. Stir the blended sweetcorn and the spinach, 5-spice and soy sauce into the pan with the rice mixture. It should have a moist, thick texture, like risotto; if it looks too dry, add a splash more water. Cook until the spinach has defrosted and heated through, then mash with the back of a fork to break down the rice grains slightly. Serve in bowls with strips of omelette on the side as finger food.

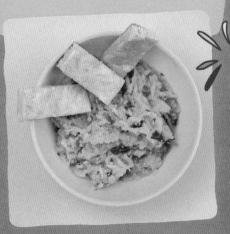

lovely leftovers!

Leftover roast pork or chicken make great additions; finely mash the meat and stir in with the spinach to heat through. You could also add flaked cooked white fish or salmon.

113

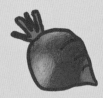

makes **36** | prep **15** mins | cook **25** mins

ruby-red mini muffins

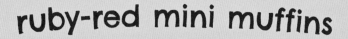

Using boppin' beetroot + crunchy carrot, these mini muffins are perfect to accompany a meal or by themselves as finger food – and they're just the right size for little hands to hold. Go on – give these gems a go!

what you need

60 g/2¼ oz **unsalted butter**, melted, plus extra for greasing

140 g/5 oz **plain flour**

½ teaspoon **bicarbonate of soda**

1 teaspoon **baking powder**

1 large **egg**, lightly beaten

150 ml/¼ pint **natural yogurt**

30 g/1 oz **feta cheese**, grated

1 small **carrot** (about 60 g/2¼ oz), peeled and grated

100 g/3½ oz **cooked beetroot** (not in vinegar), patted dry and grated

Boiled egg quarters and steamed broccoli florets, to serve

what to do

1) Preheat the oven to 190°C/375°F/Gas Mark 5. Grease 36 holes of 3 mini-muffin tins.

2) Sift the flour, bicarbonate of soda and baking powder into a large bowl and stir until combined, then make a well in the centre.

3) Beat together the egg, yogurt and melted butter in a bowl, then gradually pour into the dry ingredients and add the feta, carrot and beetroot. Using a wooden spoon, stir together gently but thoroughly until just combined.

4) Divide the mixture between the prepared muffin holes, then bake for 20–22 minutes until risen. Leave to cool slightly, then cool completely on a wire rack. Serve as finger food with boiled egg quarters and steamed broccoli florets.

our friends say...

'Finger foods saved me with baby number two! They meant I could give the little one something to hold and munch on while I fed the older one. Then I could come back to the baby to complete his meal with a puree.'

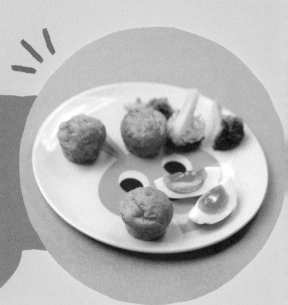

makes **12** prep **15 mins** cook **15 mins**

crispy courgette fritters

What do you get when you pair a cool courgette with frrresh herbs? A lip-smacking finger food that is just mint to be!

what you need

1 **courgette**, coarsely grated

30 g/1 oz **plain flour**

1 **egg**, lightly beaten

3 tablespoons finely grated
   Parmesan cheese

2 tablespoons very finely chopped
   mint leaves (optional)

Olive oil, for frying

**Pitta bread fingers and hummus or
   your baby's favourite dip**, to serve

what to do

1. Squeeze the grated courgette in a clean tea towel to remove any excess water, then tip it into a large bowl. Stir in the flour, egg, Parmesan and mint (if using) to make a loose batter.

2. Heat enough oil to coat the base of a large, nonstick frying pan over a medium heat. Cook the fritters – 1 heaped tablespoon of mixture per fritter – in 2 batches for 2–3 minutes on each side until light golden. Drain on kitchen paper before cutting into half-moons. Serve with pitta bread fingers and hummus or your baby's favourite dip.

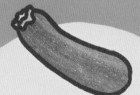

our friends say...

'I love thinking of fun ways to use food for play. One of my baby's favourites is when I use a whole courgette as a microphone. Sometimes I make him giggle by singing into it; and sometimes I use it to "interview" him about how much he loves what he's eating!'

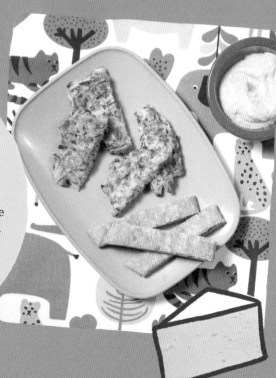

115

 serves **3–4**

 prep **15 mins**

 cook **30 mins**

grab + go cheesy eggy fingers

A cross between a tortilla + a crustless quiche, these yummy eggy fingers are crackin'! They are baked in the oven, so while you've got the oven on, why not pop in some courgette fingers to roast, too?

what you need

Olive oil, for greasing

3 **spring onions**, finely sliced

3 small **courgettes** (about 300 g/ 10$^{1}/_{2}$ oz)

4 **eggs**, lightly beaten

2 tablespoons **whole milk or milk of choice**

40 g/1$^{1}/_{2}$ oz **mature Cheddar cheese**, grated

Freshly ground **black pepper**

Your choice of **vegetables, bread, pasta or potatoes**, to serve

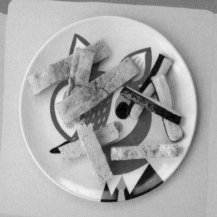

what to do

1. Preheat the oven to 180°C/350°F/Gas Mark 4. Lightly grease a 450 g/1 lb silicone loaf tin.

2. Steam the spring onions in a saucepan over a medium heat for 5 minutes or until tender.

3. Meanwhile, finely grate one of the courgettes, then wrap the grated courgette in a piece of kitchen paper or a tea towel and squeeze to remove any excess water. Cut the two remaining courgettes into sticks about the size and shape of your index finger. Toss the courgette fingers in a little oil and arrange in a small roasting tin, cover with foil and set aside until ready to cook.

4. In a large bowl, beat the eggs with the milk and season with a little pepper. Stir in the cheese and grated courgette. Mash the steamed spring onions and stir them into the egg mixture.

5. Pour the egg mixture into the prepared loaf tin. Place the loaf tin and the small roasting tin containing the courgette fingers on a baking sheet. Bake in the oven for 25 minutes, turning the courgettes over and removing the foil halfway through cooking, until the eggs have set and the courgettes are tender.

6. Carefully turn the cooked eggs out of the loaf tin and cut into 8 fingers. Serve with the roasted courgette fingers and your choice of vegetables, bread, pasta or potatoes.

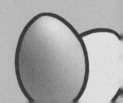

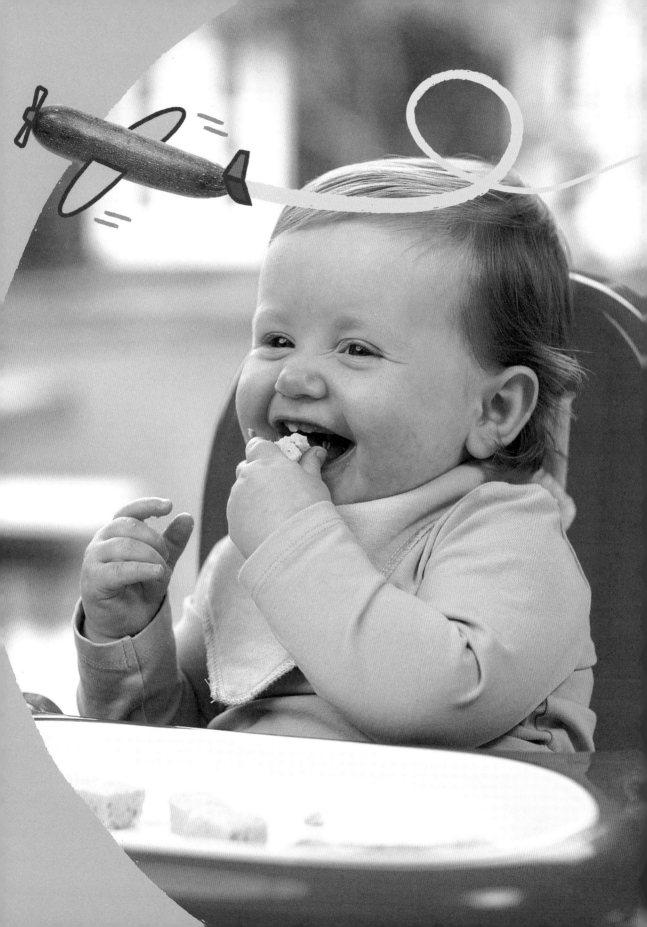

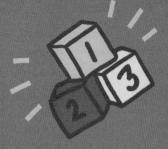

three ways with
dunky dips

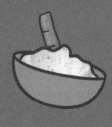

Mix + match your little one's favourite fruit or veggie dunkers with these exciting dip recipes. They're guaranteed to be a big dip!

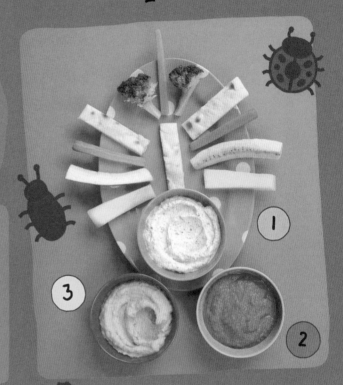

dip + dunk!

Choose from these dunkers:

☺ **Pitta bread**, cut into fingers

☺ **Vegetable sticks**, such as carrot or broccoli, cooked until very soft

☺ **Fruit sticks**, such as mango or banana, skin removed

---

① **minty cucumber + cream cheese dip**

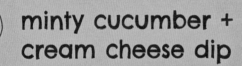

serves	prep	cook
2–3	10 mins	no cook

what you need

60 g/2¼ oz **cucumber**, roughly chopped

Handful of **mint leaves**

Juice of ½ **lemon**

4 tablespoons **cream cheese**

2–3 tablespoons **natural Greek yogurt**

1 small **garlic clove**, crushed (optional)

what to do

① Put the cucumber, mint and lemon juice in a mini food processor or blender and blend until very finely chopped or pureed.

② Tip the mixture into a bowl and stir in the cream cheese, yogurt and garlic (if using), mixing everything together. Spoon into a bowl and serve with your choice of dunkers.

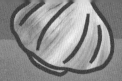

garlic bread + red pepper dip

serves 3 · prep 10 mins · cook 25 mins

what you need

2 large **red peppers**, halved, deseeded and each half cut into 4 strips, or **roasted peppers** in oil from a jar, drained

4 **garlic cloves**, unpeeled

1 tablespoon **extra virgin olive oil**, plus extra for cooking the peppers

2 slices of **bread** (about 60 g/2¼ oz), crusts removed

Juice of 1 small **lemon**

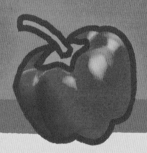

what to do

1. Preheat the oven to 200°C/400°F/Gas Mark 6. Line a baking sheet with baking parchment.

2. Put the peppers and garlic cloves on the baking sheet, drizzle with oil and turn to coat. Roast for 25 minutes, turning once, until tender. Transfer the peppers to a bowl, cover with clingfilm and let stand for 5 minutes or until cool enough to handle. If using jarred peppers you can skip this step.

3. Peel the skins off the peppers and put them in a mini food processor or blender. Squeeze the garlic cloves out of their skins and add to the peppers with the oil, bread, lemon juice and 1 tablespoon of water. Blitz until everything is smooth, adding another 1 tablespoon of water if needed. Spoon into a bowl and serve with your choice of dunkers.

sweet potato + bean dip

serves 6 · prep 5 mins + cooling · cook 10 mins

what you need

150 g/5½ oz **sweet potato**, peeled and cut into chunks

2 large **garlic cloves**, peeled

100 g/3½ oz drained **canned white beans** in water, rinsed

2 tablespoons **lemon juice**

2 tablespoons **light tahini**

1 tablespoon **olive oil**

what to do

1. Cook the sweet potato and garlic in a saucepan of boiling water for 10 minutes or until tender. Drain and leave to cool.

2. Put the sweet potato and garlic in a mini food processor or blender with the remaining ingredients and 1–2 tablespoons of water and blend until smooth and creamy, adding a splash more water if needed. Spoon into a bowl and serve with your choice of dunkers.

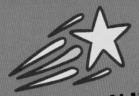

superstar sardine pasta

This sardine pasta is out of this world! Sardines are a superstar ingredient, loaded with essential omega-3s, for developing little brains + eyes!

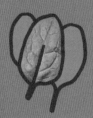

what you need

60 g/2¼ oz **dried stelline (star) pasta**

Large handful of **baby spinach leaves**, stalks removed, leaves finely chopped

125 g/4½ oz can **sardines** in water, drained and bones removed

2 teaspoons **extra virgin olive oil**

2 **tomatoes**, deseeded and diced

2 tablespoons **tomato puree**

1 tablespoon chopped **basil leaves**

Steamed broccoli florets, to serve

what to do

1. Cook the pasta in a saucepan of boiling water according to the packet instructions until tender, adding the spinach 2 minutes before the end of the cooking time. Drain, reserving the cooking water.

2. Meanwhile, mash the sardines in a bowl.

3. Heat the oil in a small saucepan over a medium–low heat and cook the tomatoes for 2 minutes or until softened. Add the tomato puree, basil, mashed sardines, cooked pasta and spinach and 4 tablespoons of the reserved cooking water and heat for 3 minutes, stirring frequently.

4. Using the back of a fork, mash the pasta mixture to a coarse puree, adding a little boiled water if necessary. Alternatively, finely chop. Serve with broccoli florets on the side as finger food.

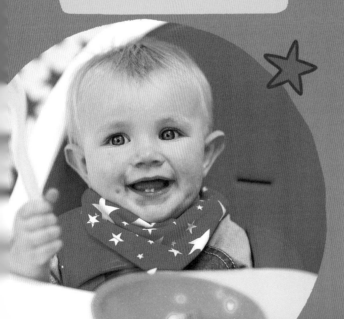
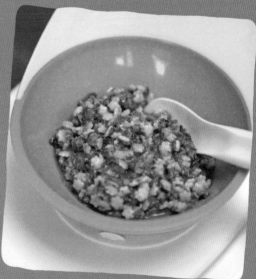

serves **3-4** prep **10** mins cook **30** mins

just-for-me VIPea salmon risotto

This risotto is fit for little VIPeas. The oregano gives it an exciting herby twist + the soft salmon is perfect for tiny teeth to practise chomping.

what you need

2 teaspoons **olive oil**

1 small **onion**, finely chopped

75 g/2¹/₂ oz **risotto rice**

¹/₂ teaspoon **dried oregano**

300 ml/¹/₂ pint hot low-salt **vegetable stock**

40 g/1¹/₂ oz **frozen petits pois**

1 small **leek**, trimmed, cleaned and finely chopped

1 tablespoon **whole milk or milk of choice**, plus extra if needed

100 g/3¹/₂ oz drained **canned wild red salmon or cooked salmon fillet** (weight without bones and skin)

what to do

1) Heat the oil in a saucepan over a medium heat. Add the onion, part-cover with a lid and cook, stirring frequently, for 5 minutes or until softened. Add the rice and oregano and stir until combined with the onion. Pour in the stock and cook, stirring frequently, for 25 minutes or until the rice is soft and the stock has been absorbed.

2) Meanwhile, steam the petits pois and leek in a saucepan over a medium heat for 4 minutes or until tender. Using a hand blender, puree the vegetables with the milk, then set aside.

3) Add the salmon and vegetable puree to the pan with the rice and heat through. Cover with a lid and leave to stand for 2 minutes.

4) Using the back of a fork, mash the rice mixture to a coarse puree, adding more milk if necessary. Alternatively, finely chop.

rice, rice, baby

If reheating the risotto after freezing, make sure you defrost it first in the fridge, then reheat thoroughly until piping hot, adding a splash of extra stock or milk.

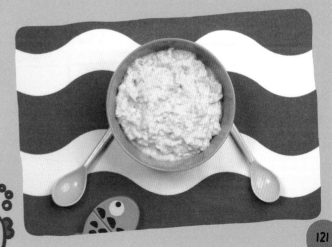

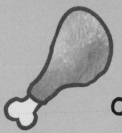

cheeky chicken croquettes

Quinoa gives these cheeky croquettes a crispy coating + the sweetcorn provides sweetness to balance the tang of the chives. Good chives only!

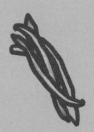

what you need

40 g/1½ oz **quinoa**, rinsed well

40 g/1½ oz **cooked chicken**, finely chopped

3 tablespoons drained no-salt, no-sugar **canned sweetcorn**, finely chopped

2 tablespoons finely chopped **chives**

½ teaspoon **unsalted butter**

Olive oil, for frying (optional)

To serve

Handful of **fine green beans**, trimmed and steamed until very soft

Flatbread, cut into strips

Dip of choice (see pages 118–119 for ideas)

what to do

1. Tip the quinoa into a small pan and pour over enough just-boiled water to cover by 2 cm/¾ inch. Return the water to the boil, then turn down the heat to low and simmer, part-covered with a lid, for 15 minutes or until the quinoa is cooked and very soft.

2. Drain the quinoa and return to the pan with the chicken, sweetcorn, chives and butter. Heat over a low heat, stirring, until warmed through, then blend briefly to a coarse paste or mash with the back of a fork, making sure the sweetcorn is broken down. Leave until cool enough to handle.

3. Divide the quinoa mixture into six pieces and press each one firmly into a croquette shape. Serve the quinoa fingers as they are or fry for a more crisp, golden coating. To fry, heat a little oil in a small frying pan and cook the quinoa croquettes for 4–5 minutes, turning occasionally, until light golden all over. Serve with steamed green beans, flatbread and a favourite dip.

rub-a-dub-dub

It's important to rinse the quinoa well under water before cooking to get rid of any bitterness in the grain.

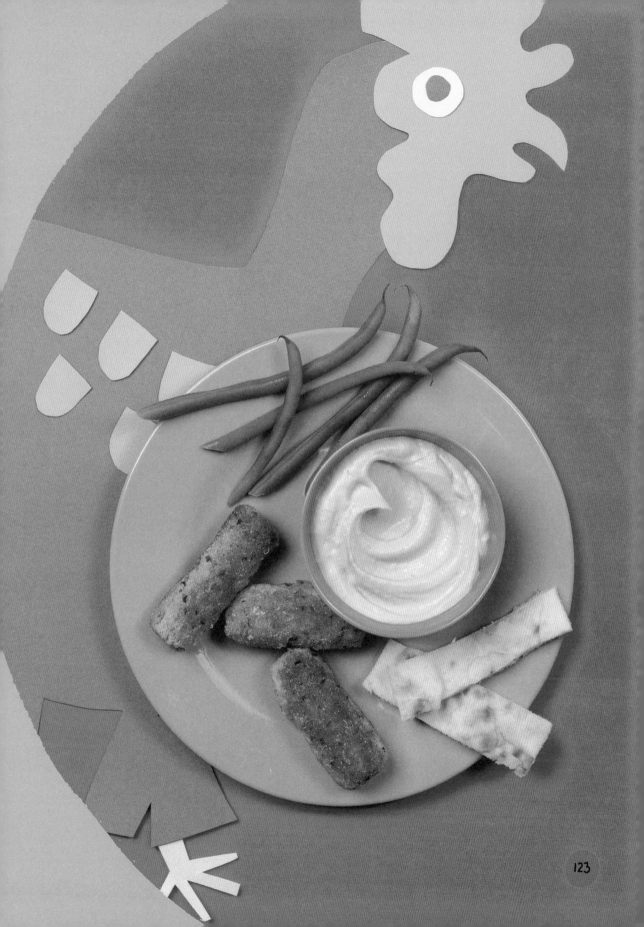

123

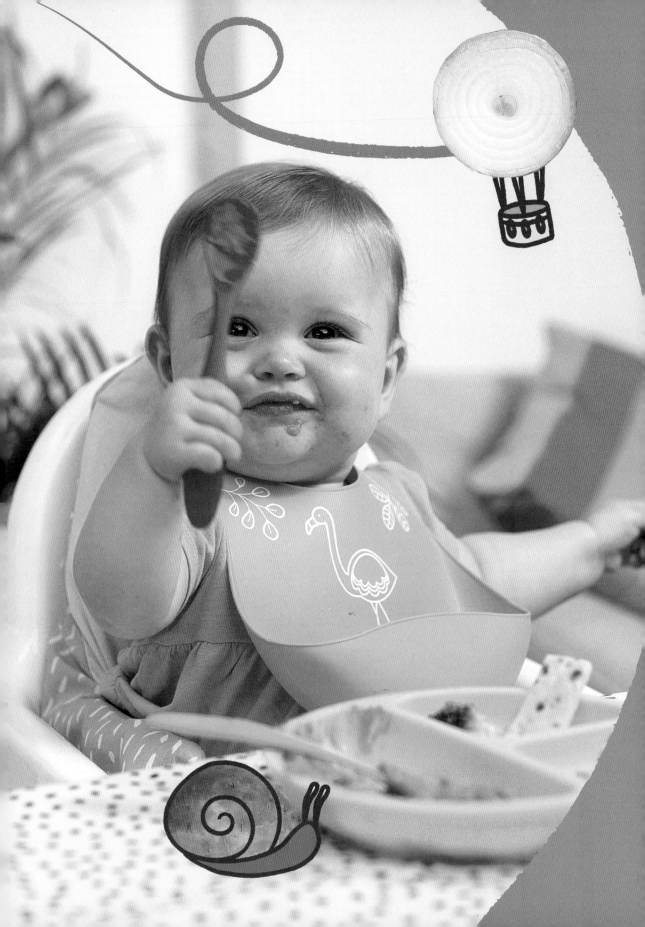

serves **2–3** | prep **15 mins** | cook **30 mins**

nuts-for-you sweet potato stew

Your little one will have nut'in but love for this sweet potato stew. Made with warming spices + tasty veg, it's a hug in a bowl!

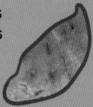

what you need

2 teaspoons **olive oil**

1 **onion**, finely chopped

60 g/2¼ oz **white cabbage**, finely shredded

1 large **garlic clove**, crushed

2 tablespoons **tomato puree**

1 teaspoon **mild smoked paprika**

2 small **sweet potatoes** (about 300 g/ 10½ oz in total), peeled and cut into 1 cm/½ inch pieces

2 teaspoons no-salt, no-sugar **peanut butter**

60 ml/2 fl oz **whole milk or milk of choice**, plus extra if needed

Squeeze of **lime juice** (optional)

Flatbread, cut into fingers, and **steamed green veg**, to serve

what to do

1. Heat the oil in a saucepan over a medium heat, add the onion and cook, stirring occasionally, for 7 minutes or until softened. Stir in the cabbage and garlic and cook for another 3 minutes, turning down the heat if the vegetables start to brown.

2. Stir in the tomato puree and paprika, followed by the sweet potatoes. Add 300 ml/½ pint of water, stir, then bring to the boil. When the sauce starts to bubble, turn the heat down and simmer, part-covered with a lid, for 15 minutes or until the sweet potatoes are tender.

3. Add the peanut butter and milk, stir and warm through briefly. Finish with a squeeze of lime (if using). Spoon into bowls and coarsely mash with the back of a fork for babies, adding more milk if needed to ensure the texture is soft and moist. Serve with fingers of flatbread and steamed green veg.

suuuper swaps!

Why not swap the sweet potatoes for butternut squash, carrot or pumpkin?

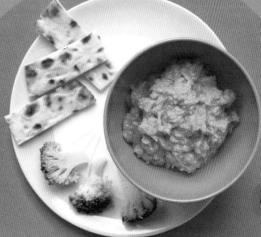

125

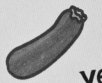

serves
4

prep
15 mins

cook
15 mins

veggie feast pasta + cheese
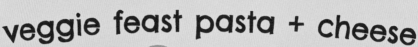

This veggie pasta feast is a real treat! Made with tiny star-shaped pasta + green veg in a cheese sauce, it's bound to get a gold-star review!

what you need

75 g/2¹/2 oz **dried stelline (star) pasta**

75 g/2¹/2 oz **cauliflower**, finely grated

1 small **courgette**, grated

1 small **leek**, trimmed, cleaned and very finely chopped

For the cheese sauce

15 g/¹/2 oz **unsalted butter**

2 teaspoons **plain flour**

250 ml/9 fl oz **whole milk or milk of choice**, warmed, plus extra if needed

¹/2 teaspoon **English mustard**

50 g/1³/4 oz **Cheddar cheese**, grated

what to do

1. Cook the pasta in a saucepan of boiling water according to the packet instructions until tender, adding the cauliflower, courgette and leek 3 minutes before the end of the cooking time. Drain, reserving the cooking water.

2. Meanwhile, make the cheese sauce. Melt the butter in a small saucepan over a low heat, add the flour and cook, stirring continuously, for 1¹/2 minutes. Gradually pour in the milk, stirring continuously, and cook for 6–8 minutes until the sauce has thickened. Remove from the heat and stir in the mustard and the cheese. Keep stirring until the cheese has melted.

3. Tip the cooked pasta and vegetables into the sauce, stir and add 2 tablespoons of the reserved cooking water if necessary.

4. Using the back of a fork, mash the pasta mixture to a coarse puree, adding a little extra reserved cooking water if necessary. Alternatively, chop it finely.

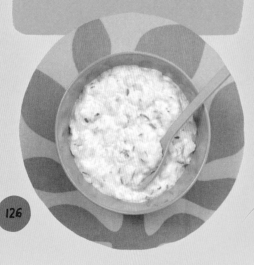
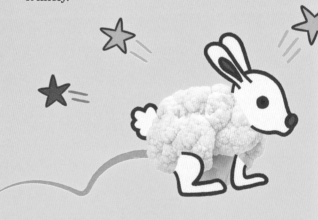

serves **2** | prep **10 mins** | cook **20 mins**

nicely spiced rice 'n' peas

Your little one will love this creamy, coconuty rice dish.
Just pop in the herbs + spice to make it reeeally nice!

what you need

2 teaspoons **olive oil**

1 small **onion**, finely chopped

30 g/1 oz **white cabbage**, grated

1 small **carrot** (about 50 g/1³⁄₄ oz),
finely grated

175 g/6 oz cooked **brown rice**

60 g/2¹⁄₄ oz drained **canned kidney
beans or borlotti beans** in water,
rinsed

¹⁄₃ teaspoon **dried thyme**

¹⁄₃ teaspoon **ground allspice**

175 ml/6 fl oz **coconut milk**

30 g/1 oz **frozen petits pois**

Handful of **green beans**, to serve

what to do

1. Heat the oil in a saucepan over a medium heat,
add the onion, cabbage and carrot and cook, part-
covered with the lid and stirring occasionally, for
8 minutes or until softened.

2. Add the cooked rice, beans, thyme, allspice and
coconut milk and stir well. Turn the heat down to
low and simmer, stirring often, for 10 minutes or
until the rice is piping hot.

3. Meanwhile, steam the petits pois and green beans
until tender (or cook them in a microwave).

4. Mash the rice and beans with the back of a fork to
a soft but still chunky texture, adding a little boiled
water if necessary. Stir in the petits pois and serve
in bowls with steamed green beans on the side as
a finger food.

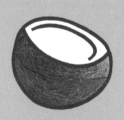

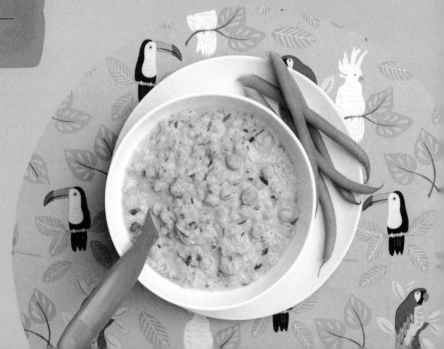

serves **3-4**
 prep **15** mins
 cook **30** mins

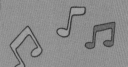

rockin' roasted squash + cashew pasta

Make tiny tums sing with this rockin' recipe.
Using veggies, herbs + pasta, it's veg,
hugs + rock 'n' roll!

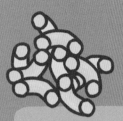
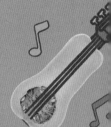

what you need

350 g/12 oz **butternut squash**,
  peeled and deseeded

1 small **onion**, cut into 6 wedges

2 **garlic cloves**, unpeeled

2 teaspoons **olive oil**

20 g/3/4 oz toasted **cashew nuts
  or blanched almonds**

100 g/3 1/2 oz **dried pasta**

1/2 teaspoon **dried thyme**

Steamed green veg, to serve

what to do

1. Preheat the oven to 200°C/400°F/Gas Mark 6.
   Cut 300 g/10 1/2 oz of the squash into 1 cm/1/2 inch
   cubes. Cut the remaining squash into 1 cm/1/2 inch
   wide fingers, about 8 cm/3 1/4 inches long.

2. Put the squash, onion and garlic in a roasting tin.
   Drizzle over the oil, toss until coated and roast
   for 30 minutes, turning once, or until tender.

3. Meanwhile, put the cashews or almonds in a
   heatproof bowl and pour over 100 ml/3 1/2 fl oz just-
   boiled water. Cover with a plate and leave to soak.

4. Cook the pasta in a saucepan of boiling water
   according to the packet instructions until tender.
   Drain, reserving 3 tablespoons of cooking water.

5. When the squash is roasted, set aside the squash
   fingers. Put the cubed squash and onion in a food
   processor or blender with the thyme and the nuts
   with their soaking water. Squeeze the garlic cloves
   out of their skins into the blender and blend,
   adding as much of the reserved cooking water as
   needed to make a smooth and creamy sauce.

6. Mash or finely chop the pasta, then stir into the
   sauce, adding a splash of the reserved water if
   needed. Serve in bowls with the fingers of squash
   and steamed green veg on the side as finger food.

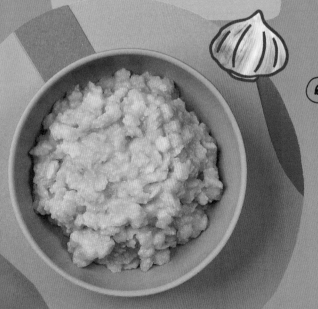

cool beans!

You could add finely shredded cooked chicken
or mashed haricot beans for extra protein.

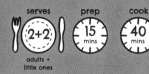

serves **2+2** adults + little ones

prep **15** mins

cook **40** mins

oh-fish-ially tasty fish fingers

Made with polenta for an extra crunchy coating + lemon zest for a citrus twist, our fish fingers are so good they have the oh-fish-ial seal of approval!

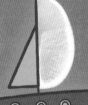

what you need

4 tablespoons **plain flour**

1 large **egg**, lightly beaten

125 g/4½ oz **instant polenta**

Finely grated zest of 1 small unwaxed **lemon**

3 thick skinless, boneless **cod or salmon fillets or other firm fish** (about 115 g/4 oz each), cut widthways into fingers 2.5 cm/ 1 inch wide

Steamed veg and Mushy Pea Dip (see page 130), to serve

For the potato wedges

2 **potatoes**, cut into wedges

Olive oil, plus extra for drizzling

what to do

1. Preheat the oven to 190°C/375°F/Gas Mark 5. Line two baking sheets with baking parchment.

2. To make the potato wedges, put the potatoes in a bowl, drizzle over enough oil to coat and toss them with your hands. Tip the potatoes on to one of the prepared baking sheets and spread out evenly. Cook the potatoes in the oven for 30–40 minutes, turning half way, until cooked through but not too crisp.

3. Meanwhile, prepare the fish fingers. Drizzle a little oil over the second baking sheet. Place the flour in a shallow dish and the beaten egg in a bowl. Place the polenta in a second shallow dish and mix in the lemon zest. Dip each fish finger into the flour, then the egg, followed by the polenta until coated. Place on the baking sheet and drizzle with more oil.

4. Fifteen minutes before the wedges are ready, place the baking sheet with the fish fingers in the oven and cook for 10–15 minutes, turning them halfway through the cooking time, until golden and cooked through. Serve the fish fingers and potato wedges as finger foods with your little one's favourite veggies and the mushy pea dip for dunking.

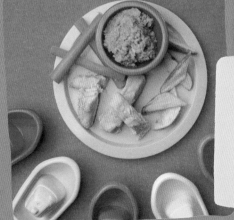

just for fun polenta pictures

The grainy texture of polenta makes it perfect for drawing pictures. Pour some polenta onto a tray (a dark-coloured tray works best) and show your little one how to use a finger to draw simple pictures in the grains.

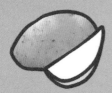

 makes **10**

 prep **20** mins

 cook **25** mins

squishy tuna fishcakes + mushy pea dip

Try these tasty, squishy little fishcakes at teatime!
They're just right for little hands to dunk, dunk, dunk
into the deeelicious mushy pea dip. You'll want to
make them at every oppor-tuna-ty!

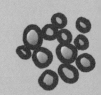

what you need

280 g/10 oz **potatoes**, cut into chunks

1 small **carrot** (about 60 g/2¼ oz), peeled and chopped

60 g/2¼ oz drained **canned tuna chunks** in spring water

1 tablespoon very finely snipped **chives**

1 teaspoon **Dijon mustard**

15 g/½ oz **unsalted butter**, melted

3 tablespoons **plain flour**, plus extra for dusting

2 tablespoons **olive oil**

For the mushy pea dip

175 g/6 oz **frozen peas**

4 tablespoons **whole milk or milk of choice**

what to do

1. Cook the potatoes in a saucepan of boiling water for 12–15 minutes until tender, adding the carrot for the last 7 minutes of the cooking time.

2. Meanwhile, make the mushy pea dip. Cook the peas in a saucepan of boiling water for 4 minutes or until tender. Drain and puree the peas with the milk in a mini food processor, or using a hand blender, until the mixture is smooth. Transfer to a bowl and set aside.

3. Drain the potatoes and carrot. Leave the potatoes to dry and cool slightly, then peel off the skins and coarsely grate into a large bowl. Using the back of a fork, mash the carrot until almost smooth. Mash the tuna and add to the bowl with the potatoes. Add the carrot, chives, mustard and melted butter, then stir well.

4. Place the flour in a shallow bowl and dust your hands with a little extra flour. Divide the potato mixture into 10 equal pieces and shape into 10 patties. Lightly dust each patty in flour until coated all over.

5. Heat the oil in a large, nonstick frying pan over a medium heat and cook the fishcakes for 3 minutes on each side until golden. Drain on kitchen paper. Serve with the mushy pea dip.

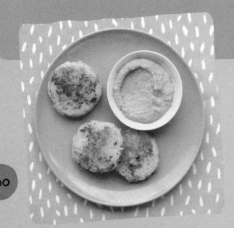

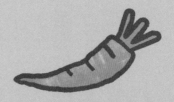

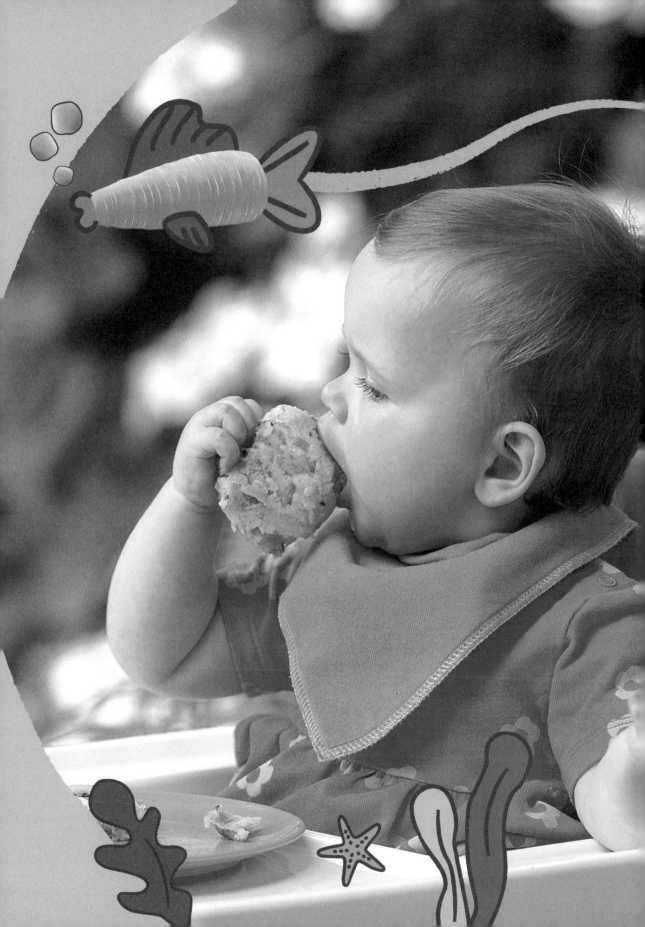

serves **3–4** · prep **10** mins · cook **25** mins

cool coconut-y lentil + turkey curry

Guaranteed to be gobbled up, this nicely spiced turkey curry uses turkey, veggies, coconut milk + lentils. Be sure to make extra for all the family!

what you need

2 teaspoons **olive oil**

125 g/4½ oz **minced turkey**, finely chopped

1 small **leek**, trimmed, cleaned and very finely chopped

1 teaspoon minced **fresh root ginger**

1 large **garlic clove**, crushed

½ small **red pepper**, cored, deseeded and finely chopped

1 teaspoon **mild curry powder**

½ teaspoon **ground turmeric**

30 g/1 oz **dried split red lentils**, rinsed

50 g/1¾ oz **frozen chopped spinach**

200 ml/7 fl oz **coconut milk**

150 g/5½ oz cooked **white basmati rice**

what to do

1. Put the oil, minced turkey, leek, ginger, garlic and red pepper in a saucepan and cook over a medium–low heat, stirring to break up any clumps of meat, for 8–10 minutes. Stir in the spices and lentils.

2. Pour 200 ml/7 fl oz of water into the pan and bring up to the boil, then turn the heat down to low and simmer, part-covered with the lid, for 10 minutes, or until the lentils are cooked.

3. Add the spinach and coconut milk and cook, stirring occasionally, for another 5 minutes or until heated through. Stir in the cooked rice and heat until piping hot, then mash with the back of a fork or blend briefly with a hand blender, adding a splash more water if needed. Leave to cool slightly before serving.

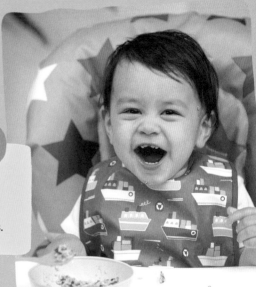

feeling hot, hot, hot!

If using leftover cooked rice, make sure you reheat it thoroughly until piping hot. Cooked rice should only be reheated once and will keep in the fridge for up to 3 days.

serves **4** | prep **15 mins** | cook **50 mins**

wonderfully warming shepherd's pie

We've spiced up this family favourite by adding cumin + ginger, plus we've included a boost of green veg, too. It's a shepherd's delight!

what you need

2 teaspoons **olive oil**

125 g/4$\frac{1}{2}$ oz **minced lean lamb**

1 small **onion**, finely chopped

1 **carrot** (about 75 g/2$\frac{1}{2}$ oz), grated

75 g/2$\frac{1}{2}$ oz **spring cabbage**, finely chopped

2 **garlic cloves**, chopped

$\frac{1}{2}$ teaspoon **ground cumin**

1 teaspoon **ground ginger**

2 teaspoons **balsamic vinegar**

1 tablespoon **tomato puree**

250 g/9 oz **sweet potatoes**, peeled and cubed

2 tablespoons **whole milk or milk of choice**

15 g/$\frac{1}{2}$ oz **unsalted butter**, cut into small pieces

what to do

1. Preheat the oven to 200°C/400°F/Gas Mark 6. Heat the oil in a saucepan over a medium heat and cook the minced lamb, breaking it up with the back of a fork, for 5 minutes or until browned all over. Remove the mince using a slotted spoon and set aside on a plate.

2. Pour off all but 2 teaspoons of the oil in the pan, then add the onion, carrot and cabbage and cook, stirring frequently, for 8 minutes or until softened. Reduce the heat slightly and stir in the garlic, then return the mince to the pan with the cumin, ginger, vinegar, tomato puree and 150 ml/$\frac{1}{4}$ pint boiled water and stir well. Cover with a lid and cook for 15 minutes or until cooked through.

3. Meanwhile, cook the sweet potatoes in a saucepan of boiling water for 10–15 minutes until tender, then drain and return to the pan. Add the milk and mash until smooth.

4. Spoon the lamb mixture into a small ovenproof dish and top with the mash. Dot the butter on top and bake in the oven for 20 minutes or until starting to crisp on top.

5. Using the back of a fork, mash the shepherd's pie to a coarse puree, adding a little boiled water if necessary. Alternatively, finely chop.

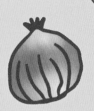

gimme-gimme beefy stew

This hearty beefy stew will warm little tums + keep them full to fuel their adventures. Gimme! Gimme! Gimme!

what you need

2 teaspoons **olive oil**

125 g/4$\frac{1}{2}$ oz **minced beef**

1 small **onion**, grated

75 g/2$\frac{1}{2}$ oz **white cabbage**, grated or finely chopped

1 small **courgette** (about 100 g/3$\frac{1}{2}$ oz), grated

1 **garlic clove**, grated

150 g/5$\frac{1}{2}$ oz drained **canned haricot, cannellini or butter beans** in water, rinsed

1 teaspoon **dried oregano**

4 **cloves**

2.5 cm/1 inch piece of **cinnamon stick** or $\frac{1}{2}$ teaspoon **ground cinnamon**

400 g/14 oz can **chopped tomatoes**

175–200 ml/6–7 fl oz low-salt **vegetable stock**

2 tablespoons **natural Greek yogurt**

Steamed broccoli florets and mashed potato or pitta bread, cut into fingers, to serve

what to do

1. Heat the oil in a saucepan over a medium heat, add the minced beef and cook, stirring, for 5 minutes or until browned. Remove the mince using a slotted spoon and set aside on a plate.

2. Reduce the heat slightly and add the onion, cabbage, courgette and garlic and a splash of water if needed, then stir to combine. Cover the pan with a lid and cook, stirring often, for 5 minutes or until softened.

3. Return the mince to the pan with the beans, oregano, cloves, cinnamon, tomatoes and stock. Reduce the heat to low, cover with a lid and simmer, stirring occasionally, for 20 minutes or until the vegetables are tender and the mince is cooked. Discard the cloves and cinnamon, if using a stick.

4. Mash the stew with the back of a fork, adding a splash of water if needed, to a coarse puree. Leave to cool slightly, then serve in bowls with a spoonful of yogurt. Serve with steamed broccoli florets and mashed potato or pitta bread fingers.

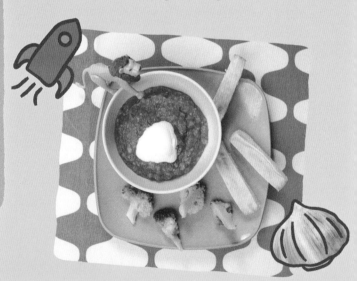

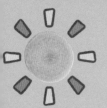

serves **2–3**

prep **10 mins**

cook **20 mins**

golden sunshine chicken

Taste the sunshine with this super-speedy, veg-licious dish, which uses golden turmeric + crunchy carrot for a pop of colour!

what you need

2 teaspoons **olive oil**

1 small **onion**, finely chopped

2 **garlic cloves**, chopped

75 g/2¹/₂ oz **cauliflower**, finely grated

75 g/2¹/₂ oz **basmati rice**, rinsed

200 ml/7 fl oz low-salt **chicken stock**

1 **carrot** (about 75 g/2¹/₂ oz), peeled and sliced

100 g/3¹/₂ oz **cooked chicken**, finely chopped

¹/₂ teaspoon **ground turmeric**

15 g/¹/₂ oz **unsalted butter**

Favourite **steamed green veg**, to serve (optional)

what to do

1. Heat the oil in a saucepan over a medium–low heat. Add the onion and cook for 6 minutes, stirring frequently. Add the garlic and cook, stirring occasionally, for another 1 minute or until softened.

2. Stir the cauliflower and rice into the pan. Pour in the stock and 100 ml/3¹/₂ fl oz water and stir well. Bring to the boil, then reduce the heat to its lowest setting, cover with a lid and simmer for 10 minutes or until the rice is tender – there should be some liquid left in the pan.

3. Meanwhile, in a saucepan over a medium heat, steam the carrot for 5 minutes or until tender. Puree the carrot with 1 tablespoon of boiled water in a food processor, or using a hand blender.

4. Stir the cooked chicken, turmeric and butter into the rice mixture and heat through thoroughly. Stir in the carrot puree, cover with a lid, and leave to stand for 2 minutes.

5. Using the back of a fork, mash the rice mixture to a coarse puree, adding a little extra boiled water if necessary. Alternatively, finely chop. Serve with your favourite steamed green veg, if you like.

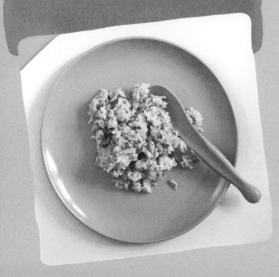

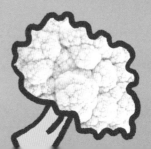

135

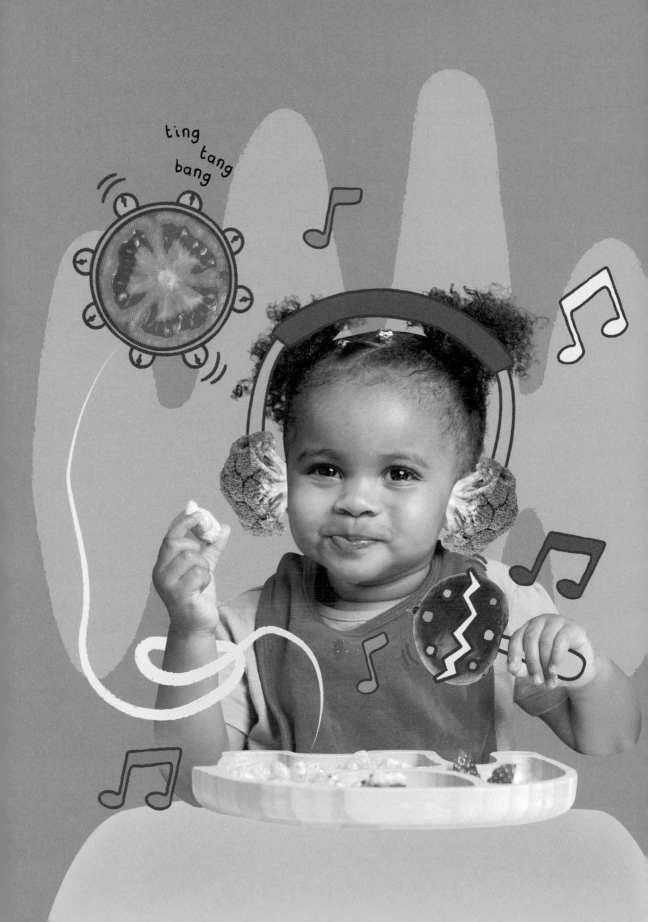

ting
tang
bang

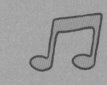

from
12
months

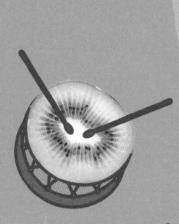

at the big table

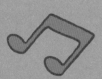

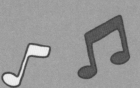

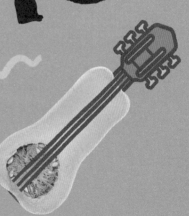

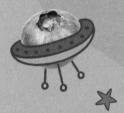

from 12 months

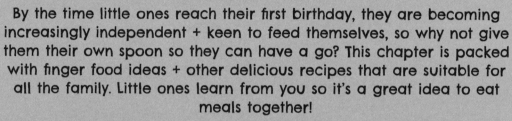

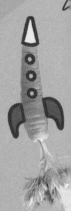

By the time little ones reach their first birthday, they are becoming increasingly independent + keen to feed themselves, so why not give them their own spoon so they can have a go? This chapter is packed with finger food ideas + other delicious recipes that are suitable for all the family. Little ones learn from you so it's a great idea to eat meals together!

what to give

While toddlers grow a bit more slowly than babies, they're often more active and, as they still have teeny tiny tummies, it's best to keep them topped up by offering three meals plus two nutritious snacks a day, and milk (see opposite for tips on milk). You can also offer a small dessert after some meals if you wish. This is a great way to include more fruit and yogurt in your little one's diet and we have some yummy recipes for you to try, too, such as Cheeky Cherry Custard Pud or Oh-so-fruity Yogurt Pots (see pages 198 and 199).

Snacks help boost energy and nutrients to keep little bodies growing and active. They can be like mini meals and contribute to the 5-5-3-2 food group recommendations below. For example, a snack portion of pitta fingers, hummus and cucumber sticks would deliver a carb, protein and veg food, while a pot of natural yogurt with berries would provide a dairy food and a fruit portion.

Try to offer the following each day from meals and snacks and remember to include lots of variety to keep things interesting, fun and provide a wide range of nutrients.

☺ 5 starchy carb foods (examples are rice, bread, potatoes, pasta and grains like oats, quinoa)

☺ 5 vegetables or fruits in a rainbow of colours

☺ 3 portions of dairy foods (milk, yogurt, cheese or fortified, no-added-sugar dairy-free alternatives)

☺ 2 portions of protein foods or 3 portions if the little one is vegetarian or vegan (meat, fish, pulses like lentils and beans, eggs or soya products like tofu and meat alternatives)

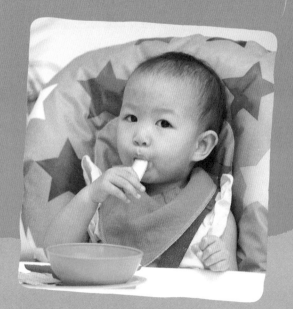

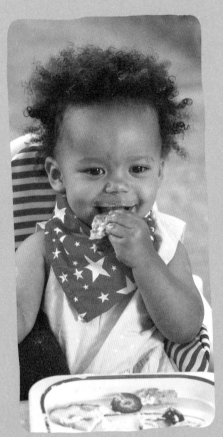

tips on texture

By the age of 12 months, lots of little ones have quite a few teeth and some might even have some molars coming through. They are now much better at chewing and moving soft pieces of food round in the mouth. Those with front teeth will now be better at biting off chunks of food and, as molars come through (around the age of 12–18 months), they'll be able to chew firmer and more fibrous foods better too. Little ones are getting more handy and can now use simple cutlery and pick up small, soft pieces like soft fruit chunks with more dexterity. But remember, every little one is different and they'll develop at their own pace.

Meals don't have to be served in a puree or sauce anymore as long as the chunks are soft and squishable under a fork and cut into small pieces (about 1 cm/ 1/2 inch cubes are ideal). Finger foods can now be a wider range of shapes rather than just batons, as long as they're still soft and easy to fit into little hands. It's still advisable to avoid hard, fibrous, stringy, flaky, gristly or brittle textures to minimize choking risks. Here are some preparation tips to keep foods a nice safe texture:

☺ Cook meat and fish so they're still moist, finely chop or mash and check for bones and any tough or gristly bits; only serve as a finger food if very soft with no gristle or bones

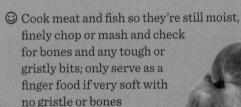

☺ Grate hard foods like raw carrot or apple

☺ Chop round foods like grapes, cherry tomatoes or sausages into quarters lengthways

☺ Avoid biscuits, bars and snacks that crumble into hard pieces or hard cereals that are served just with milk

milky newsflash

You can breastfeed your little one for as long as you like. If your baby has been having formula as a main drink, you can now switch to whole or semi-skimmed cows' milk and offer around 350 ml/12 fl oz a day. Wait until your little one is 5 years old before giving skimmed milk as it's too low in calories to fuel their growth. If your baby is dairy-free, go for a fortified, no-added-sugar milk alternative with added calcium, iodine and vitamins B12 and D.

creating a healthy relationship with food

Food refusal (either turning up their noses at new foods or rejecting foods that have previously been accepted) is really common among toddlers and is a completely normal part of their development so try not to take it personally – it's not your cooking skills!

Unfortunately, healthy foods like green veg taste bitter and other foods can be squishy or slimy, like banana. While the rejection response might once have been protective against eating poisonous foods, it now is more likely to result in a big 'NO!' to broccoli.

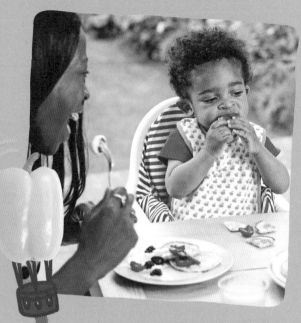

Food refusal doesn't mean your toddler is fussy or picky, though. It's a normal part of development so try not to stress. But some little ones can become fussy, and this is, in part, due to genetics, which is why some will be pickier than others.

Food refusal and fussiness can be a phase that begins around the age of 2 years and may persist for many years. Fortunately, there are lots of things you can do to navigate this tricky period and avoid mealtime battles.

Lots of research shows that repeatedly offering a rejected food can help little ones to become more familiar and eventually accept it. This can take 15–20 separate experiences of that food though, so you might want to make a note of how many times you've offered that food on a tracker.

This sounds like a lot of wasted food and mealtime stress but remember, an experience of a food doesn't necessarily mean it has been tasted. It can be touching a raw piece of broccoli, helping with the cooking, even if the food doesn't go on their plate, or putting the food to their lips without tasting it. That's why sensory play outside of mealtimes can be so powerful. See pages 20–21 for more information.

Here are some top tips for creating happy little eaters:

☺ **Role model good eating behaviour** If your toddler sees you, their siblings or friends eating a food they have rejected or are wary of, they might feel happier to give it a try. Eating together as a family when you can is great for showing toddlers how it's done, without too much pressure!

☺ **Serve food family style** This means putting food in the middle of the table and letting little people serve themselves (with a bit of help). You choose what's offered (and you can pop cooking dishes and saucepans straight on the table without transferring to bowls to save on washing up if you like). It's up to your toddler to decide what they choose and how much of it to eat. That way, they can see a disliked food on the table, but they don't feel they have to eat it. It still counts as an experience of that food.

☺ **This or that?** Like family-style serving, if you give your toddler a choice of two or three veggies to go on the plate and encourage everyone to pick one or two, your toddler can feel in control of what they're eating, while still being exposed to a variety of foods.

☺ **Pop a side plate next to your toddler's main plate** If your toddler decides they don't want to eat a food, they can pop it on the side plate. There's no pressure to eat the food but when they put it to one side, they're interacting with it and therefore increasing their familiarity, even without eating it.

☺ **Offer a rejected food in different forms** Instead of boiling or steaming veg, try stir-frying or roasting them; instead of cooked carrot, offer it raw and finely grated.

tingling taste buds

Keep strong tastes on the menu but try to avoid foods with any added salt and steer clear of lots of added sugar. Toddlers can now safely eat honey so they can occasionally enjoy it as a sweet treat, for example in our Best-of-the-bunch Banana Muffins (see page 200).

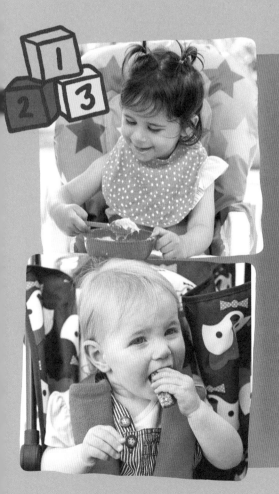

how much?

It's still really important to trust your little one's appetite and let them tell you when they've had enough (see page 17). As adults, we might 'find room' for dessert or eat when we're sad or bored but little ones don't do that unless we show them how! Let them respond to their appetite. If you find they refuse their dinner because they're waiting for dessert then try serving both at the same time. Even if they eat pudding first and then their meal, that's OK!

Refer to the portion size guide on page 99 for tips on how much to serve – little hands get bigger as toddlers get older so they're still a great reference point for serving sizes! Serve small portions to begin with, as little ones can be put off by a large plate of food, and offer second helpings.

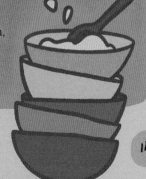

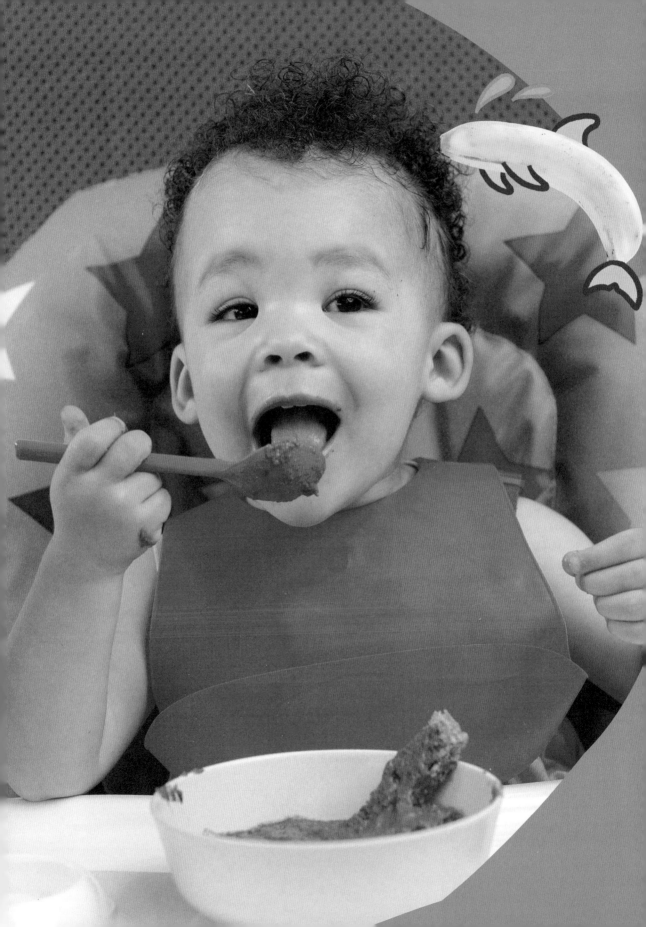

serves **2**
 prep **10 mins**
 cook **no cook**

all-in-one smoothie bowl

This super smoothie bowl is just what you want on a hot summer's day. Defrost your cherries overnight, or use partly defrosted for a cooool bowl.

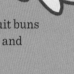

what you need

150 g/5½ oz **frozen dark pitted cherries**, defrosted or semi-defrosted

1 small **banana**, peeled and halved

1 small cooked **beetroot** (not in vinegar), quartered

4 tablespoons **natural Greek yogurt**

1½ tablespoons **rolled oats**

1 teaspoon **ground mixed seeds**

¼–½ teaspoon **ground cinnamon**

½ teaspoon **vanilla extract**

Lightly toasted buttered fruit buns or bread, cut into fingers, to serve

what to do

1. Place all the ingredients, except the fruit buns or bread, in a food processor or blender and puree until thick, smooth and creamy.

2. Pour or spoon the smoothie into bowls and serve with fingers of lightly toasted fruit bun or bread.

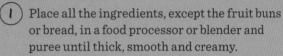

suuuper swaps

Use 40 g/1½ oz frozen chopped spinach, defrosted, in place of the beetroot and cherries, and replace the small banana with a large banana.

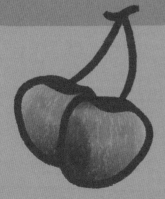

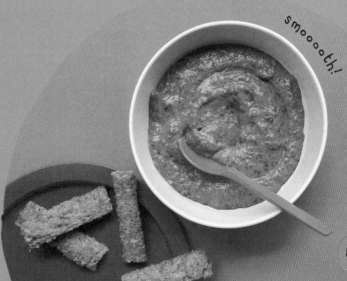

smooooth!

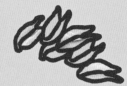

super seeds brekkie bars

Just the right size + shape for little hands to hold, these brekkie bars are great whether you are at home or on the go. Once the mixture is chilled, simply cut into fingers + enjoy!

what you need

100 g/3½ oz **porridge oats**

50 g/1¾ oz **pecan nuts**

3 tablespoons **ground mixed seeds**

175 g/6 oz unsulphured **dried apricots**, roughly chopped

75 g/2½ oz **raisins or dates**

4 tablespoons **fresh orange juice**

Natural yogurt, to serve

what to do

1. Line an 18 cm/7 inch square baking tin with baking parchment. Place the oats in a large, nonstick frying pan and dry-fry over a medium–low heat, tossing frequently, for 5–6 minutes until golden and crisp. Tip into a large mixing bowl and leave to cool.

2. Add the nuts to the pan and dry-fry over a medium–low heat for 3–4 minutes, turning once, until golden. Tip into a separate bowl and leave to cool.

3. Press the toasted oats between your fingers to crush them slightly. In a food processor or blender, whiz the pecans until coarsely chopped and then add to the bowl with the oats. Stir in the ground mixed seeds until everything is combined.

4. Place the apricots, raisins or dates and orange juice in a food processor or blender and blend to a smooth, thick puree. Scrape the fruit puree into the bowl with the dry ingredients and mix well until combined.

5. Spread the fruit mixture in an even layer, about 1 cm/½ inch thick, in the prepared baking tin. Chill for 1 hour or until firm. Cut into 18 bars and store in a lidded container in the fridge – they will keep for up to 5 days. Serve with some natural yogurt for dunking.

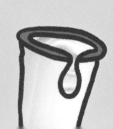

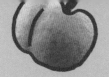

serves **4**

prep **20 mins** + chilling

cook **no cook**

cheeky peachy cheesecake pots

Who said you can't have dessert for brekkie?
Pair juicy peach + sweet carrot for a tasty start
to the day! Peach-perfect!

what you need

410 g/14½ oz can **peach slices** in natural juice, drained and chopped

1 small cooked **carrot** (about 60 g/ 2¼ oz), chopped

100 g/3½ oz **cream cheese**

50 ml/1¾ fl oz **natural Greek yogurt**

1 teaspoon **vanilla extract**

For the cheesecake base

4 **oatcakes**, roughly broken

1 tablespoon **ground mixed seeds**

½ teaspoon **ground cinnamon**

1 teaspoon **clear honey or maple syrup**

1 tablespoon melted **unsalted butter**

what to do

1. To make the cheesecake base, blitz the oatcakes in a mini food processor or blender to fine crumbs, then tip into a bowl and stir in the ground seeds, cinnamon, honey or maple syrup and butter until combined. Spoon 1½ tablespoons of the oat mixture into each of 4 small glasses or ramekins, lightly pressing it down with the back of a spoon into an even layer.

2. Put the peach and cooked carrot in a food processor or blender and blend to a smooth puree, then set aside.

3. In a bowl, beat together the cream cheese, yogurt and vanilla. Spoon the cream cheese mixture on top of the oatcake base in the glasses or ramekins. Top with the peach puree, then chill until ready to serve. For babies, mix everything together until combined before serving.

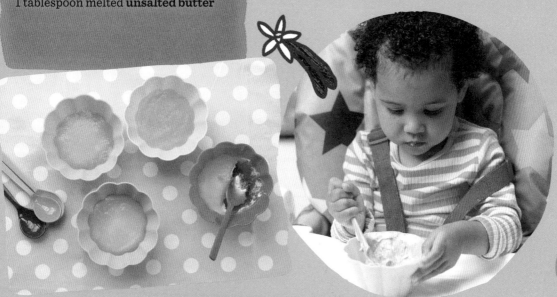

three ways with
toast toppers

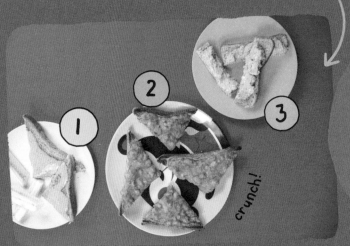

crunch!

The perfect speedy brekkie, toast doesn't need to be boring. Why not try these tasty toast toppers for some easy ways to add fun new tastes to your little one's mornings?

(1) nut butter drizzle
with banana toasts

serves **2-4**   prep **10 mins**   cook **5 mins**

what you need

100 g/3½ oz toasted **unsalted skinless hazelnuts** (or use toasted unsalted peanuts or cashews)

1 teaspoon **ground cinnamon**

5 tablespoons **whole milk or milk of choice**

1 teaspoon **vanilla extract**

2 teaspoons **sunflower oil**

2 slices of your favourite **bread**

1 **banana**, peeled and sliced or mashed

what to do

(1) Finely grind the hazelnuts in a mini food processor. Add the cinnamon, milk, vanilla extract and oil and process again for about 5 minutes, occasionally scraping down the sides, until you have a smooth and creamy nut butter.

(2) Meanwhile, toast the bread in the toaster.

(3) Spread some of the nut butter over each slice of toast in an even layer. (Put any remaining nut butter in a lidded container and store in the fridge for up to 5 days.) Top with the banana, then cut each piece into quarters or fingers to serve.

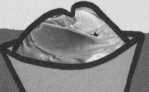

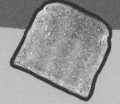

② cheesy beans on garlic toast

 serves **2–4** prep **5** mins cook **10** mins

what you need

2 slices of your favourite **bread**

100 g/3½ oz drained **canned haricot or cannellini beans** in water, rinsed

1 tablespoon **tomato puree**

30 g/1 oz **mature Cheddar cheese**, grated

½ teaspoon **mild smoked paprika**

1 **garlic clove**, peeled and halved (optional)

Unsalted butter, for spreading

what to do

① Preheat the grill to high. Toast one side of each slice of bread.

② Meanwhile, using the back of a fork, mash the beans well in a bowl, then stir in the tomato puree, cheese and paprika.

③ Remove the toast from the grill and (if using) rub the cut side of the garlic clove over the untoasted side of the bread. Spread the butter over the same side, then top with the bean mixture, spreading it out evenly to the edges. Place the toasts under the grill for 5 minutes or until the cheese has melted. Leave until cool then cut into quarters.

③ eggy pesto toasts

 serves **2–4** prep **5** mins cook **10** mins

what you need

2 **eggs**

1 small **avocado**, halved, stoned and flesh scooped out

2 teaspoons **mayonnaise**

3 teaspoons **green or red pesto**

2 slices of your favourite **bread**

what to do

① Cook the eggs in a saucepan of boiling water for 8 minutes or until hard boiled. Drain and run under cold running water, then peel off the shells. Roughly chop into small pieces.

② Mash the avocado in a bowl with the back of a fork until smooth. Add the mayonnaise, pesto and chopped eggs and mash again until very finely mashed.

③ Meanwhile, toast the bread in the toaster, then spread the egg mixture evenly over the top of the toast. Cut into fingers to serve.

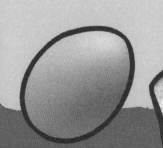

crackin' creamy eggs

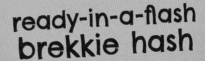

serves 2+2 adults + little ones   **prep** 5 mins   **cook** 15 mins

4 tablespoons drained no-sugar, no-salt **canned sweetcorn** or 100 g/3¹/₂ oz **frozen chopped spinach**, defrosted and mashed slightly with the back of a fork

8 **cherry tomatoes**, diced

4 **eggs**

4 teaspoons **crème fraîche**

30 g/1 oz **Cheddar cheese**, grated

Bread, toasted, to serve

what to do

1. Preheat the oven to 180°C/350°F/ Gas Mark 4. Divide the sweetcorn or spinach and diced cherry tomatoes between 4 large ramekins.

2. Crack an egg into each ramekin, on top of the vegetables. Top the eggs with 1 teaspoon of the crème fraîche and a sprinkling of cheese.

3. Place the ramekins on a baking sheet and bake in the oven for 15 minutes or until set. Leave to cool slightly and either serve in the ramekins (if the ramekins are cool enough to hold) or spoon into bowls. Serve with fingers of toast.

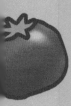

ready-in-a-flash brekkie hash

serves 2+2 adults + little ones   **prep** 10 mins   **cook** 10 mins

1¹/₂ tablespoons **olive oil**

300 g/10¹/₂ oz **cooked potatoes**, cut into small chunks

2 **cooked carrots**, cut into small chunks

150 g/5¹/₂ oz **cooked cabbage**, cut into small pieces

140 g/5 oz **cooked sprouts**, sliced

4 **tomatoes**, diced

1 teaspoon **mild smoked paprika**

2 teaspoons **garlic powder**

2 tablespoons **tomato puree**

4 **hard-boiled eggs,** shelled and cut into sixths

what to do

1. Heat the oil in a large frying pan over a medium heat. Add the potatoes and cooked vegetables and stir-fry for 5 minutes or until everything is starting to turn golden.

2. Add the tomatoes, spices and tomato puree and cook for another 3 minutes or until the tomatoes break down. Add a splash of water to the pan if it seems dry. Serve the hash with the hard-boiled eggs on the side and fingers of toast.

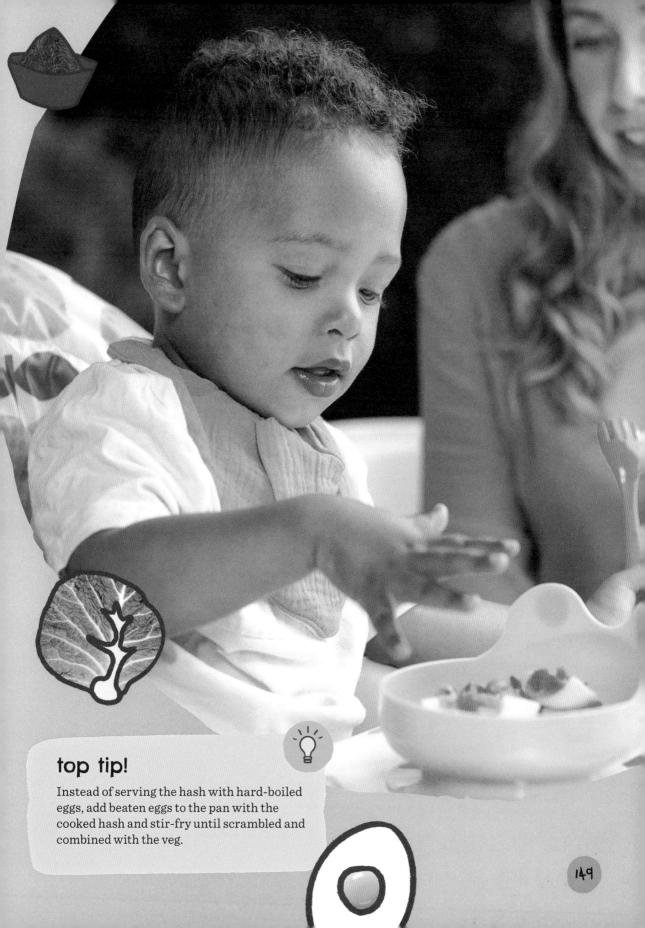

top tip!

Instead of serving the hash with hard-boiled eggs, add beaten eggs to the pan with the cooked hash and stir-fry until scrambled and combined with the veg.

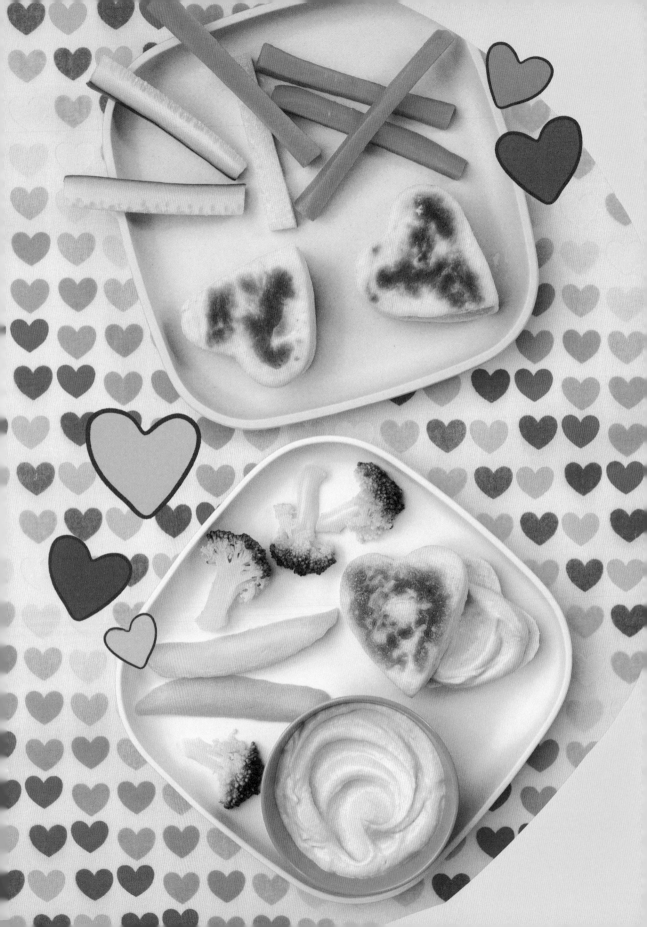

makes 10   **prep** 10 mins   **cook** 10 mins

from 12 months

lovely hearts brekkie bread rolls

You don't have to be a baker to whisk up these brekkie rolls. With just a few simple ingredients, all you 'knead' is 10 minutes to prep the dough + then you can get creative with your shapes! We've suggested hearts for some luuurve to start your day!

what you need

200 g/7 oz **plain flour**, plus extra for dusting

1 rounded teaspoon **baking powder**

1/2 teaspoon **salt**

100 ml/31/2 fl oz **whole milk or milk of choice**

2 tablespoons **natural yogurt**

1 tablespoon **vegetable oil**

Serving ideas

Sweet or savoury spreads

Cheese, cut into fingers

Steamed vegetable or fruit sticks

Scrambled, poached or hard-boiled egg

Hummus or other dip

Grilled tomatoes and mushrooms

what to do

1 Sift the flour, baking powder and salt into a mixing bowl and make a well in the middle.

2 Mix together the milk, yogurt and oil in a jug, then pour into the dry ingredients. Using a fork, mix everything together until combined, then form into a ball of dough with your hands. Do not over-mix the dough or it will become tough.

3 Tip the dough out of the bowl on to a lightly floured work surface. Using a rolling pin, roll the dough out until about 1 cm/1/2 inch thick. Stamp out 10 hearts with a heart-shaped cutter, re-rolling the dough when needed.

4 Heat a large nonstick frying pan, with a lid, over a medium heat. Arrange the hearts in the pan (you may need to cook them in two batches) and turn the heat to medium–low. Cover the pan with the lid and cook for 9–10 minutes, turning once or twice, until light golden and risen. Serve warm with your choice of filling or finger foods.

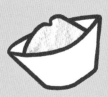
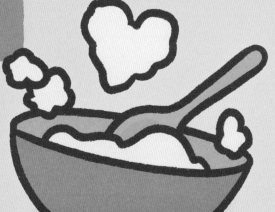

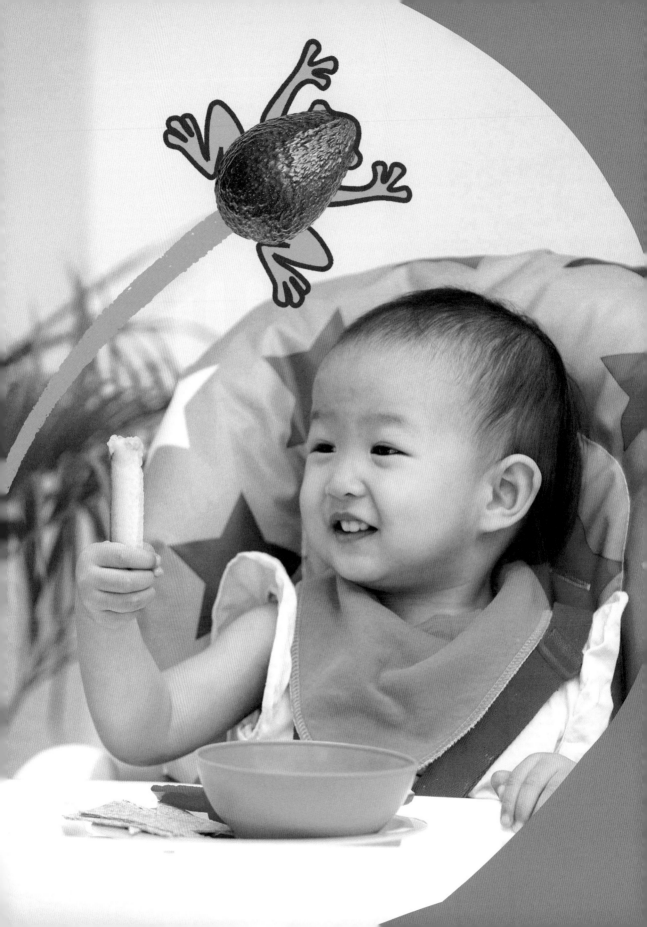

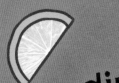

serves **2** · prep **10 mins** · cook **5 mins**

dippy pea guacamole

Chunks of avocado can slip + slide when small hands try to pick them up. To make it easier for your little one, mash the avocado with some peas + serve the dip with veggie sticks! Go on, avo' go!

what you need

60 g/2¼ oz **frozen petits pois**

1 small **avocado**, halved and stoned

2 teaspoons **lime or lemon juice**

6 tablespoons **baby's usual milk**

A few **fresh coriander leaves**, finely chopped (optional)

To serve

2 small low-salt soft **wholemeal tortillas**, cut into fingers

Steamed vegetable sticks

what to do

1. Steam or boil the petits pois in a small saucepan over a medium heat for 3–4 minutes until tender. Drain, if necessary, and tip into a bowl.

2. Scoop out the avocado flesh into the bowl and pour in the citrus juice and milk. Using the back of a fork, mash together until almost smooth. Alternatively, puree using a hand blender.

3. Stir in the coriander (if using). Serve the guacamole with the tortilla fingers and steamed vegetable sticks for dunking.

our friends say...

'Some slippery foods, such as banana or avocado, were really tricky for my little one to pick up. So, I would coat the pieces in wheatgerm (which is nutritious, too!) to make them easier for his little hands to grasp hold of.'

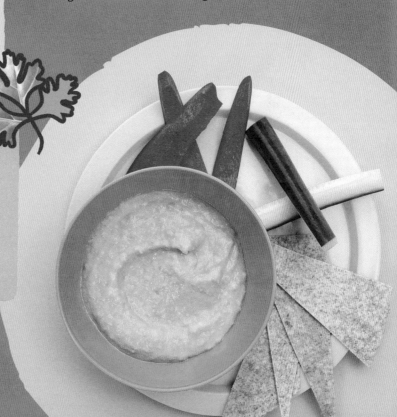

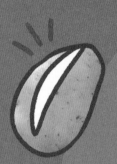

three ways with baby baked potatoes

Baked potatoes are an easy + nutritious mealtime fave! Our tasty fillings are quick to put together, so you can prep them while the potatoes are baking. Then, once the potato is ready, just scoop the fluffy insides out, mash in the filling + serve in a bowl.

baby baked potatoes

serves **2** prep **5 mins** cook **1 hour**

what you need

2 small **potatoes** (about 125 g/4½ oz each), scrubbed

Filling (see opposite) and **favourite vegetables**, to serve

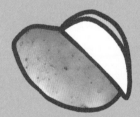

what to do

1. Preheat the oven to 200°C/400°F/Gas Mark 6. Place a skewer through each potato to speed up the cooking time, then bake in the oven for about 1 hour or until cooked through.

2. When the potatoes are ready, cut each one in half and finely chop the skin and potato, mashing the flesh with the back of a fork until almost smooth. Add your chosen filling and mash together. Serve with some favourite veg.

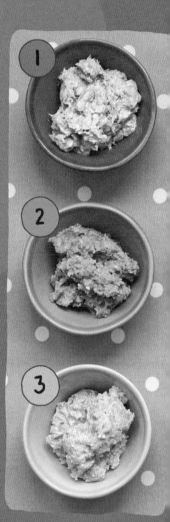

tuna, cheese + chive filling

serves **2** | prep **5 mins** | cook **no cook**

what you need

85 g/3 oz drained **canned tuna chunks** in spring water

2 tablespoons **cream cheese**

3 tablespoons **natural yogurt**

2 tablespoons snipped **chives**

what to do

1. Mash the tuna chunks in a bowl and mix in the cream cheese, yogurt and chives.

---

pea + pesto filling

serves **2** | prep **5 mins** | cook **5 mins**

what you need

200 g/7 oz **frozen peas**

4 teaspoons **red or green pesto** (see box, page 83)

2 teaspoons **olive oil**

20 g/3/4 oz **Cheddar cheese**, finely grated

what to do

1. Steam or boil the peas in a saucepan over a medium heat for 3 minutes or until tender.

2. Put the cooked peas, pesto, olive oil and 1–2 tablespoons of boiled water in a food processor, or use a hand blender, and puree until almost smooth. Stir in the cheese.

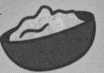

---

chicken + vegetable filling

serves **2** | prep **10 mins** | cook **10 mins**

what you need

2 **carrots**, thinly sliced

6 tablespoons drained no-salt, no-sugar **canned sweetcorn**

6 tablespoons **natural yogurt**

60 g/2¼ oz **cooked chicken**, finely chopped

what to do

1. Steam or boil the carrots in a saucepan over a medium heat for 6–8 minutes until tender.

2. Put the cooked carrots, sweetcorn, yogurt and 1–2 tablespoons of boiled water in a food processor or blender and whiz to a coarse puree. Stir in the chicken.

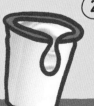

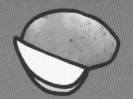
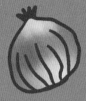

serves **2+2** adults + little ones | prep **15** mins | cook **30** mins

pizza-ta-ta-ta

What do you get if you cross a pizza with a frittata? This super-tasty pizza-ta-ta-ta, of course! Get little noses to sniff, sniff, sniff the fresh basil!

what you need

150 g/5½ oz **potatoes**, peeled and quartered

1 tablespoon **olive oil**

1 large **onion**, diced

2 **garlic cloves**, finely chopped

1 teaspoon **dried oregano**

6 **eggs**, lightly beaten

85 g/3 oz **mozzarella cheese**, torn into pieces

4 teaspoons **red or green pesto** (see box, page 83)

5 **cherry tomatoes**, halved

Handful of **pitted black olives** (not in brine), quartered

Some torn **basil leaves** (optional)

Steamed **vegetable sticks**, to serve

what to do

① Steam or boil the potatoes in a saucepan over a medium heat for 12–15 minutes until tender. Drain, if necessary, and leave to cool slightly, then cut into small chunks.

② Meanwhile, heat the oil in a nonstick, ovenproof frying pan over a medium heat. Cook the onion, stirring frequently, for 8 minutes or until softened. Stir in the garlic and oregano and cook for a further 1 minute.

③ Preheat the grill to medium–high. Pour the eggs into the pan with the onion, add the potatoes, pressing them down into the egg mixture, and cook over a medium–low heat for 8 minutes or until the base is set and light golden.

④ Scatter over the cheese and dot with the pesto. Top with the tomatoes, olives and basil (if using), then grill for 3–4 minutes until the cheese has melted and the egg is cooked. Leave to stand for 1–2 minutes before cutting into wedges, or fingers for babies. Serve with steamed vegetable sticks.

top toppings!

Why not experiment with different toppings such as sliced mushrooms, sweetcorn, steamed broccoli florets, chopped red pepper or spinach?

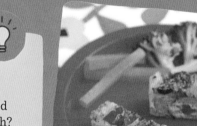

serves **1+2** adults + little ones

 prep **10** mins

 cook **15** mins

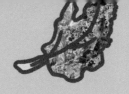

sizzle-sizzle tomato-y scramble

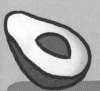

This tasty twist on scrambled eggs uses tomatoes, red peppers + eggs for an unbeatable combo!

what you need

4 teaspoons **olive oil**

1 small **onion**, diced

1/2 **red pepper**, cored, deseeded and finely diced

2 **tomatoes**, deseeded and finely diced

2 teaspoons **tomato purée**

Large pinch of **dried oregano**

4 **eggs**, lightly beaten

Freshly ground **black pepper**

Cucumber sticks and warm flatbreads, cut into strips, to serve

what to do

1. Heat half of the oil in a large nonstick frying pan over a medium heat. Stir in the onion and red pepper and cook for 6 minutes or until very soft.

2. Add the tomatoes, tomato puree and oregano and cook for another 4 minutes, stirring, adding a splash of water if the mixture looks dry. Season with a little black pepper.

3. Move the tomato mixture to one side of the pan and turn the heat down to low. Pour the remaining oil into the empty side of the pan, then tip in the beaten eggs. Cook the eggs, stirring gently, for 1 1/2–2 minutes until scrambled. Stir the scrambled eggs into the tomato mixture until combined. Serve with sticks of cucumber and flatbread.

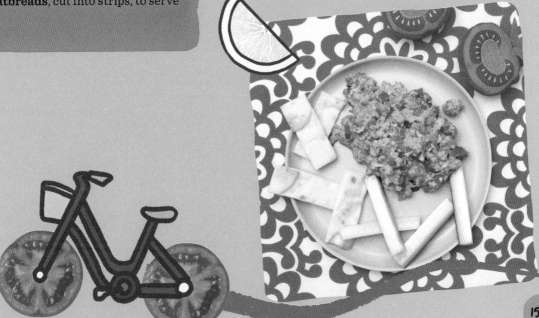

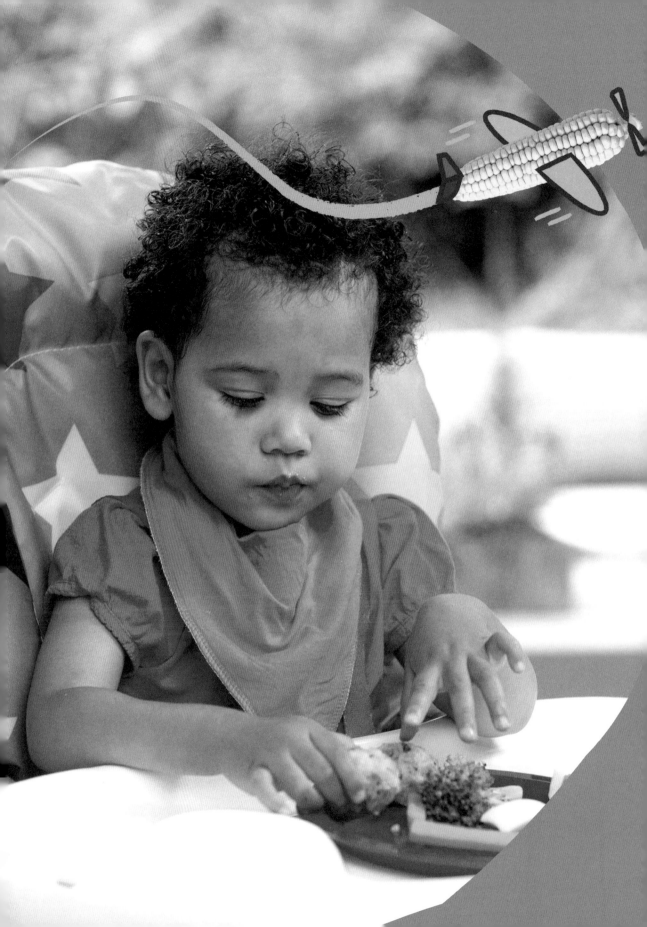

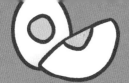

makes **16**

prep **15** mins

cook **15** mins

big + strong muffins

Burstin' with big tastes, these muffins use spinach, cheese + a little bit of mustard to pack a tasty punch!

what you need

50 g/1¾ oz **unsalted butter**, melted, plus extra for greasing

150 g/5½ oz **self-raising flour**

1 teaspoon **baking powder**

1 teaspoon **English mustard powder**

50 g/1¾ oz **baby spinach leaves**, stalks removed, and leaves very finely chopped

100 g/3½ oz drained no-salt, no-sugar **canned sweetcorn**

30 g/1 oz **mature Cheddar cheese**, finely grated

125 ml/4 fl oz **whole milk or milk of choice**

1 **egg**, lightly beaten

Hard-boiled eggs, quartered, and **steamed broccoli or vegetable sticks**, to serve

what to do

1. Preheat the oven to 190°C/375°F/Gas Mark 5. Grease 16 holes of 1 or 2 mini-muffin tins.

2. Sift the flour, baking powder and mustard powder into a large bowl. Stir in the spinach, sweetcorn and cheese until fully combined, then make a well in the centre.

3. Beat together the milk, egg and melted butter in a jug, then gradually pour into the dry ingredients and gently stir together with a wooden spoon until just combined.

4. Divide the mixture evenly between the prepared muffin holes, then bake the muffins in the oven for 12–15 minutes until risen and golden. Cool on a wire rack. Serve warm or cold with the hard-boiled eggs and steamed broccoli or vegetable sticks.

our friends say...

'I loved telling my little ones why food was good for them – "Spinach makes you really strong!" and "Milk and cheese give you superhero bones and gnashy teeth!" It's good for them to know that food isn't just about filling hungry tummies.'

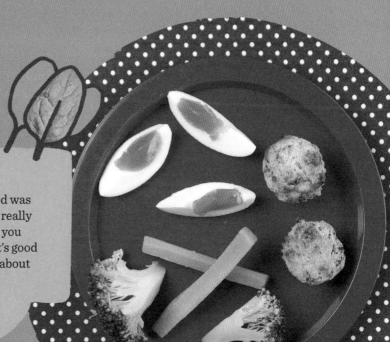

three ways with
polenta

A great alternative
to pasta, polenta is made from
cornmeal + can be used in lots of different
ways. Here are three different ideas for making
mealtimes fun, from yummy tastes to exciting shapes!
Set polenta will keep for up to 3 days in the fridge.

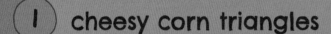

1 cheesy corn triangles

serves 2+2 adults + little ones
prep 15 mins + cooling
cook 25 mins

what you need

Olive oil, for greasing and cooking

100 g/3½ oz drained no-salt, no-sugar **canned sweetcorn**

115 g/4 oz **instant polenta**

30 g/1 oz **unsalted butter**

30 g/1 oz **Parmesan cheese**, finely grated

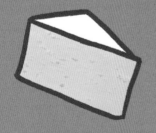

what to do

1. Lightly oil a small baking tin. Puree the sweetcorn in a food processor or blender until smooth and set aside.

2. Pour 575 ml/19 fl oz just-boiled water into a saucepan and place over a medium–low heat. Gradually pour in the polenta and cook, stirring continuously with a balloon whisk then a wooden spoon, for 8–10 minutes until smooth and thick.

3. Stir in the butter, Parmesan and pureed corn until combined. Spoon the polenta mixture into the baking tin and spread it out into an even layer, about 1 cm/½ inch thick, using a wet palette knife. Leave the polenta to cool and set. When ready to serve, cut the polenta into triangles – it should make about 18.

4. Pour enough oil into a large nonstick frying pan to cover the base and place over a medium heat. Working in batches, fry the polenta pieces for 2–3 minutes on each side until light golden and slightly crisp. Place on a kitchen paper-lined plate to drain and leave to cool slightly before serving.

2 spinach polenta chips

serves **2+2** adults + little ones

prep **15** mins + cooling

cook **25** mins

what you need

Olive oil, for greasing and cooking

115 g/4 oz **instant polenta**

30 g/1 oz **unsalted butter**

75 g/2½ oz **frozen chopped spinach**, defrosted

30 g/1 oz **Parmesan cheese**, finely grated

what to do

1. Lightly oil a small baking tin. Prepare the polenta as in step 2 of the recipe opposite.

2. Stir in the butter, spinach and Parmesan until combined.

3. Spoon the polenta mixture into the baking tin and spread it out into an even layer, about 1 cm/½ inch thick, using a wet palette knife. Leave to cool and set. When ready to serve, cut the polenta into 5 cm/2 inch long chips – it should make about 25.

4. Cook the polenta chips as in step 4 of the recipe opposite.

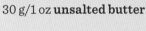

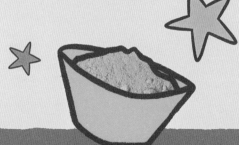

golden stars

serves **2+2** adults + little ones

prep **15** mins + cooling

cook **25** mins

what you need

Olive oil, for greasing and cooking

115 g/4 oz **instant polenta**

1 teaspoon **ground turmeric**

2 teaspoons **mild curry powder**

2 teaspoons **garlic powder**

30 g/1 oz **unsalted butter**

what to do

1. Lightly oil a small baking tin. Prepare the polenta as in step 2 of the recipe opposite.

2. Stir in the spices and butter until combined.

3. Spoon the polenta mixture into the baking tin and spread it out into an even layer, about 1 cm/½ inch thick, using a wet palette knife. Leave the polenta to cool and set. When ready to serve, use a star-shaped cutter to stamp out polenta stars – it should make about 18, depending on the size of your cutter.

4. Cook the polenta stars as in step 4 of the recipe opposite.

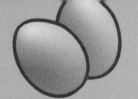

chomp-chomp cauli cheese bites

These cheesy cauli bites will have your little one chomp, chomp, chomping! The perfect size for little hands to hold, they're easy cheesy!

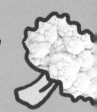

what you need

60 g/2¼ oz **cauliflower florets**, finely grated

165 g/5¾ oz cold **cooked risotto rice**

30 g/1 oz **Parmesan cheese**, finely grated

1 **egg**, lightly beaten

30 g/1 oz fresh day-old **breadcrumbs**

Olive oil, for drizzling

Serving ideas

Cooked sliced **chicken or fish strips**

Hard-boiled egg, quartered

Tomato Sauce (see page 169)

Cucumber and red pepper sticks

Hummus or other dip

what to do

1) Preheat the oven to 200°C/400°F/Gas Mark 6. Line a baking sheet with baking parchment.

2) Steam the cauliflower in a saucepan over a medium heat for 4 minutes or until tender, then cool under cold running water and drain well.

3) Place the cold cooked risotto rice in a mixing bowl and mash lightly with the back of a fork to crush the grains, then stir in the cooked cauliflower and Parmesan until combined. With wet hands, shape the mixture into 8 balls, about the size of a golf ball. (The balls can be made a few hours ahead and chilled in the fridge until ready to cook.)

4) Put the beaten egg in a shallow dish and the breadcrumbs on a plate. Using one hand, dunk a rice ball into the egg to cover and then use your other hand to coat it with the breadcrumbs. Place the coated rice ball on the prepared baking sheet and repeat to coat the remaining rice balls.

5) Lightly drizzle some oil all over the balls and then cook in the oven for 15–20 minutes, turning once, until golden and crisp and the rice is piping hot inside. Leave to cool slightly before serving halved or quartered with your choice of accompaniment.

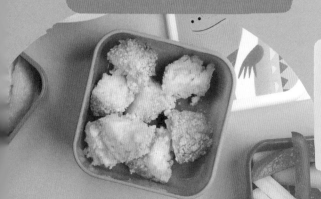

risott-oh yeah!

If cooking the risotto rice from scratch, you'll need 75 g/2½ oz risotto rice and 400 ml/14 fl oz water. Cook the rice according to the packet instructions, then let it cool completely before using.

serves **2+2** adults + little ones

prep **10** mins

cook **25** mins

super-duper chick-chick pasta

Packed with four different veggies, this super-duper dish will be the star of your little one's mealtime!

what you need

1 tablespoon **olive oil**

1 **onion**, finely chopped

2 **carrots**, finely diced

1 **celery stick**, finely diced

175 g/6 oz drained **canned cannellini beans** in water, rinsed

500 ml/18 fl oz hot low-salt **chicken stock**

1 tablespoon **tomato puree**

1 teaspoon **dried oregano**

1 **bay leaf** (optional)

2 handfuls of **kale leaves**, stalks removed, very finely chopped

150 g/5½ oz **cooked chicken**, cut into very small pieces or finely shredded

150 g/5½ oz **cooked stelline (star) pasta** (about 75 g/2½ oz uncooked weight)

Freshly ground **black pepper**

Finely grated **Parmesan cheese**, to serve (optional)

what to do

1. Heat the oil in a saucepan over a medium heat, add the onion, carrots and celery and cook, part-covered with a lid and stirring often, for 7 minutes or until softened.

2. Add the beans and stock, then stir in the tomato puree, oregano and bay leaf (if using). Bring the sauce to the boil, then turn the heat down and simmer, part-covered with a lid, for 13 minutes. Add the kale, cooked chicken and pasta, season with a little pepper and simmer for another 5 minutes or until the vegetables are tender.

3. Serve in bowls, using a fork to mash the beans and veg for babies and adding more stock to loosen if needed. Sprinkle over some Parmesan (if using).

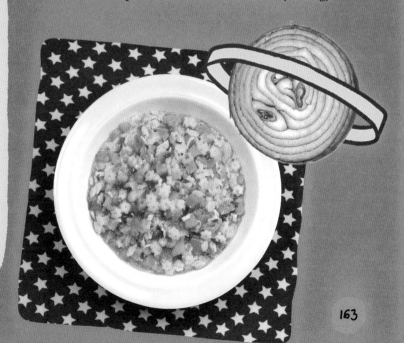

serves
2+2
adults +
little ones

prep
10 mins

cook
15 mins

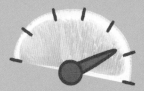

goin' goin' gone! green pasta

This delicious green pasta uses avocado, kale + basil for a yummy creamy sauce. It's so tasty, it will be goin' goin' gone before you know it!

what you need

300 g/10½ oz **dried pasta**

100 g/3½ oz **kale leaves** (weight without the stalks)

2 large **garlic cloves**, peeled

1 large **avocado**, halved, stoned and flesh scooped out

2 tablespoons **extra virgin olive oil**

Juice of **1 lemon**

Handful of **basil leaves**

Finely grated zest of ½ **unwaxed lemon**

20 g/¾ oz **Parmesan cheese**, finely grated, plus extra to serve

3 tablespoons **toasted pine nuts or favourite nut**, finely chopped (optional)

Freshly ground **black pepper**

what to do

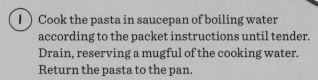

1. Cook the pasta in saucepan of boiling water according to the packet instructions until tender. Drain, reserving a mugful of the cooking water. Return the pasta to the pan.

2. Meanwhile, steam the kale and whole garlic cloves in a saucepan over a medium heat for 5 minutes or until tender, then refresh under cold running water until cool.

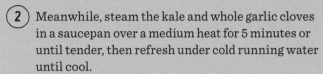

3. Put the kale, garlic, avocado, oil, lemon juice, basil leaves and 4 tablespoons of the reserved cooking water in a food processor or blender and blend until smooth and creamy.

4. Spoon the green sauce into the pan with the pasta. Stir in the lemon zest and Parmesan, then season with a little pepper. Warm through briefly, adding an extra 2 tablespoons of reserved cooking water if needed. Serve in bowls, finely chopping the pasta for babies, with extra Parmesan and the finely chopped nuts scattered over the top (if using).

power up!

For a protein boost, stir 75 g/2½ oz canned cannellini beans into the sauce when you add it to the pasta.

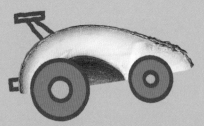

164

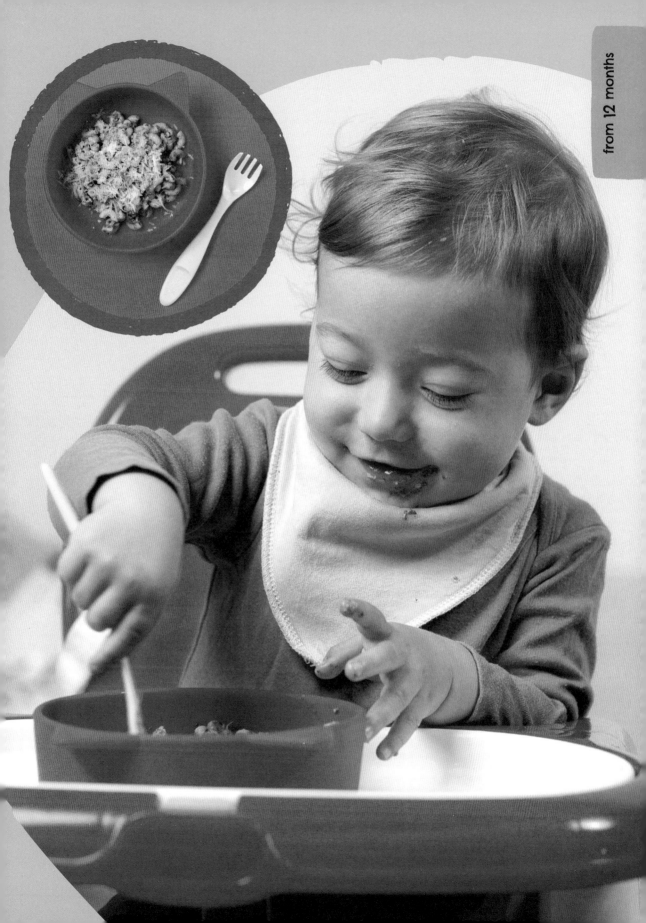

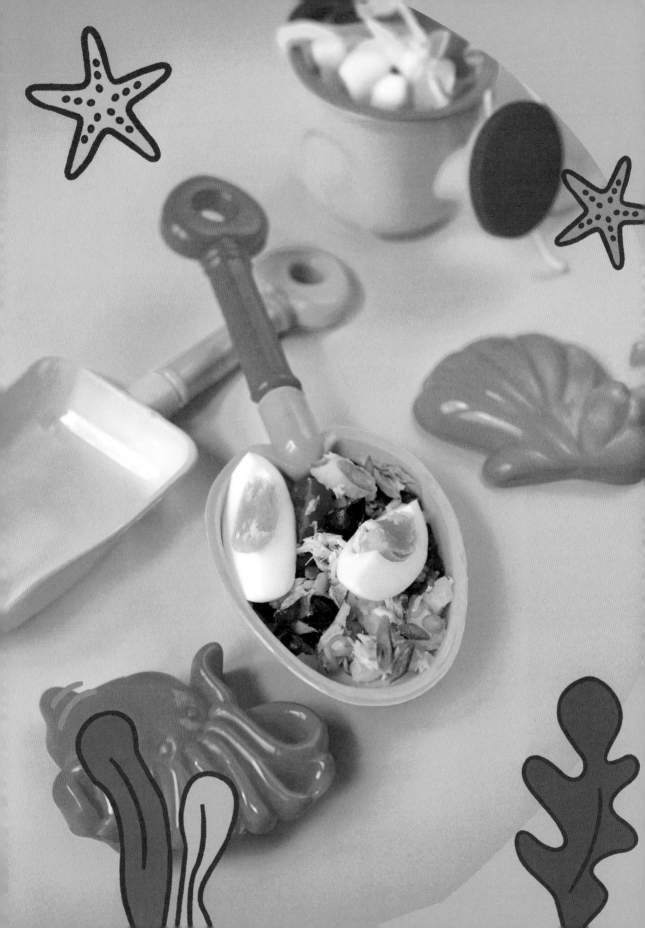

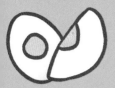

serves **1+2** adults + little ones | prep **15** mins | cook **15** mins

   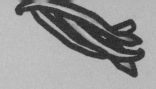

mighty mackerel salad

Perfect for filling little – and big – tums, this tasty salad is full of goodness; the tomatoes contain vitamin C, the mackerel supplies omega-3 + the eggs provide protein. Let your little one get their hands on and taste each ingredient, one by one!

what you need

280 g/10 oz **new potatoes**, halved

3 **eggs**

50 g/1¾ oz **green beans**, trimmed and very thinly sliced diagonally

140 g/5 oz **cherry tomatoes**, quartered

40 g/1½ oz **pitted black or green olives** (not in brine), halved

110 g/3¾ oz **canned grilled mackerel fillets**, skin and bones removed and flesh flaked

For the dressing (optional)

4 teaspoons **extra virgin olive oil**

4 teaspoons **lemon juice**

2 tablespoons **natural yogurt**

what to do

1) Cook the potatoes in a saucepan of boiling water for 12–15 minutes until tender, adding the eggs 10 minutes and the green beans 5 minutes before the end of the cooking time. Drain, then cool the beans and eggs under cold running water. Peel off the potato skins, if you prefer.

2) Cut the potatoes into bite-sized pieces and place in a serving bowl with the beans, tomatoes, olives and mackerel. Turn gently until combined. Shell the eggs and cut into wedges, then place next to the salad.

3) For the dressing (if using), mix together the oil and lemon juice in a small bowl until combined, then stir in the yogurt. Spoon it over the salad before serving. Finely chop the salad for babies, or serve as finger food without the dressing.

stir it up!

The sooner little ones can start to help in the kitchen, the better! See if your baby will help you to stir the dressing, then pour it over the salad.

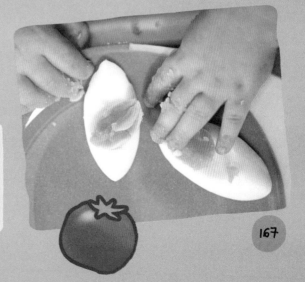

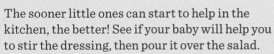

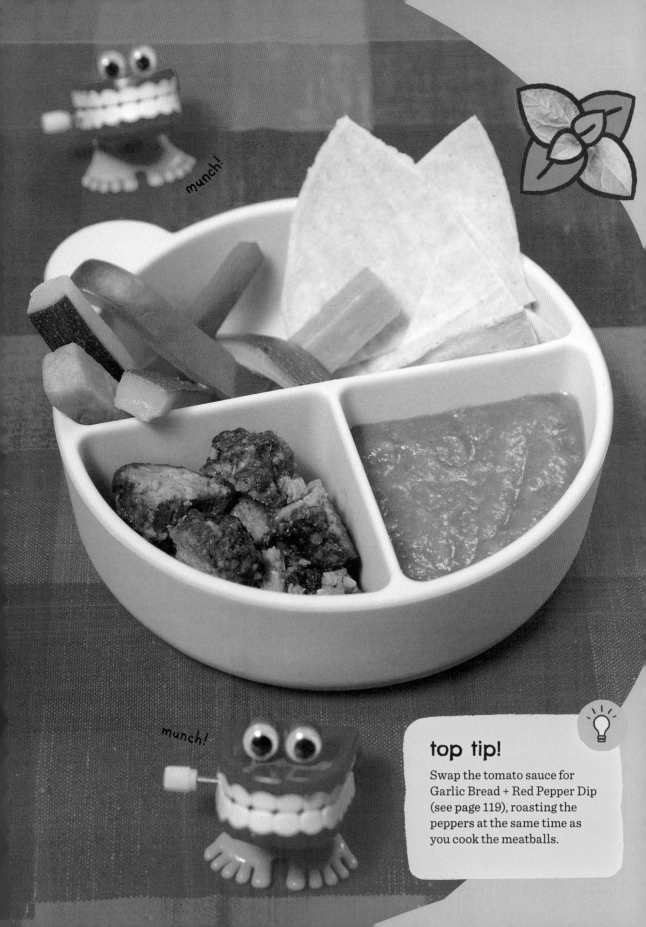

munch!

munch!

top tip!

Swap the tomato sauce for
Garlic Bread + Red Pepper Dip
(see page 119), roasting the
peppers at the same time as
you cook the meatballs.

serves **3** | prep **15 mins** + chilling | cook **20 mins**

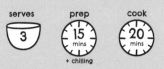

munch-munch meatballs

These cheesy, herby meatballs, which are baked in the oven + served with a roasted tomato sauce, couldn't be easier to make. Your little one will munch them all up with big slurpy smiles!

what you need

1 teaspoon **Dijon mustard**

1 small **egg**, lightly beaten

250 g/9 oz **minced beef**, finely chopped

1 **spring onion**, very finely chopped

1 large **garlic clove**, crushed

40 g/1½ oz fresh day-old **breadcrumbs**

1 teaspoon **dried oregano**

10 g/½ oz **Parmesan cheese**, finely grated

Olive oil, for brushing and drizzling

Freshly ground **black pepper**

Vegetable fingers and warm soft corn tortillas, cut into sixths, to serve

For the tomato sauce

4 **tomatoes**, quartered

1 small **onion**, quartered

1 teaspoon **tomato puree**

what to do

1. Line a baking sheet with baking parchment. Put the mustard and egg in a mixing bowl and stir with a fork to combine. Add the minced beef, spring onion, garlic, breadcrumbs, oregano, Parmesan and a little black pepper and stir until combined. Divide the mixture into 10 walnut-sized portions and shape into balls. Place the meatballs on the prepared baking sheet, cover and put in the fridge for 15 minutes, or until ready to cook, to firm up slightly.

2. Preheat the oven to 200°C/400°F/Gas Mark 6. Just before cooking, brush the meatballs with oil. Bake in the oven for 18–20 minutes, turning once, until cooked through and slightly golden.

3. Meanwhile, make the tomato sauce. Put the tomatoes and onion in a small roasting tin, drizzle over some oil and roast in the oven for 20 minutes, turning once, until tender. Transfer to a food processor or blender and blend, adding the tomato puree and a splash more oil or water, if needed, until smooth.

4. Cut the meatballs into quarters and serve as finger food with the tomato sauce, vegetable fingers and warm tortilla triangles. Alternatively, mash the meatballs with the back of a fork.

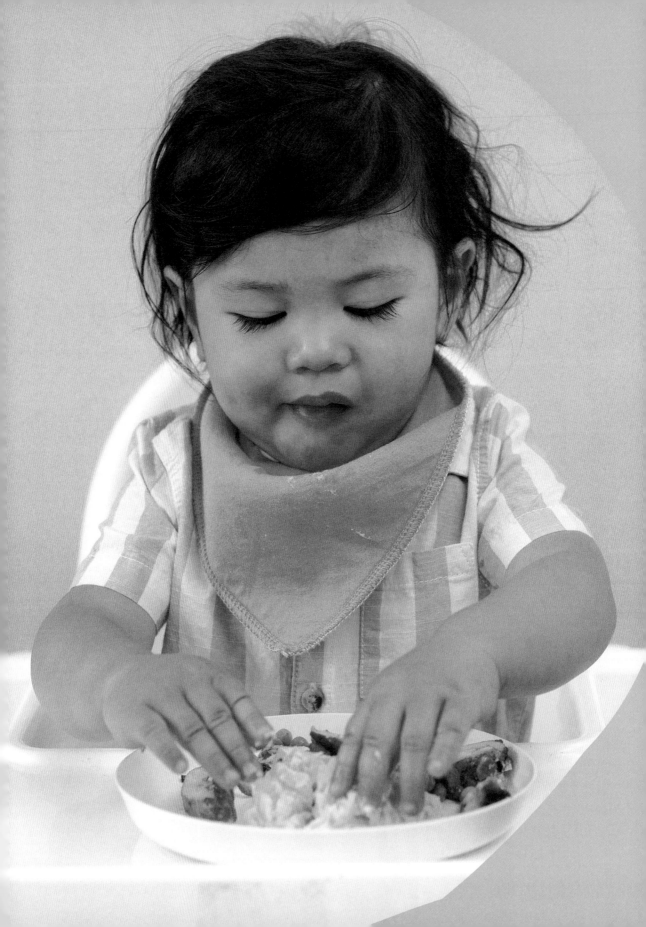

serves 2+2 adults + little ones

prep 15 mins + marinating

cook 30 mins

bangin' BBQ chicken with minty potato salad

Enjoy the yummy taste of BBQ chicken without the barbecue. Perfect for summer evenings, this dish is un-grill-ievable!

what you need

2 teaspoons **balsamic vinegar**

1 teaspoon reduced-salt **soy sauce**

1 tablespoon **tomato puree**

1 tablespoon **clear honey**

2 teaspoons **olive oil**

6 skinless, boneless **chicken thighs**

Steamed vegetables, such as peas, to serve

For the potato salad

400 g/14 oz **new potatoes**, such as Charlotte, scrubbed, halved or quartered if large

1 **spring onion**, chopped

Handful of **mint leaves**

1 **mini cucumber** (about 60 g/ 2¼ oz), chopped

1 tablespoon **natural Greek yogurt**

2 tablespoons **mayonnaise**

2 teaspoons **lemon juice**

what to do

1. In a large shallow dish, mix together the balsamic vinegar, soy sauce, tomato puree, honey and 1 teaspoon of the oil to make a marinade for the chicken. Make three cuts along the top of each chicken thigh, then place them in the dish and spoon the marinade over until coated. Cover and leave to marinate in the fridge for at least 30 minutes.

2. Preheat the oven to 200°C/400°F/Gas Mark 6. Line a roasting tin with baking parchment or foil. Place the chicken in the prepared tin, spooning over any marinade left in the dish. Cover the tin with foil and roast the chicken in the oven for 15 minutes. Remove the foil, spoon over any juices in the tin and return to the oven for another for 10–15 minutes until the chicken is cooked and golden and there is no trace of pink in the middle.

3. Meanwhile, make the potato salad. Cook the potatoes in a saucepan of boiling water for 15 minutes or until tender. To make the dressing, blend the spring onion, mint and cucumber to a coarse puree in a food processor or blender, then mix in the yogurt, mayonnaise, lemon juice and the remaining oil. Drain the potatoes well and cut into bite-sized pieces. Tip the potatoes into a serving bowl, pour the dressing over and stir gently to mix everything together.

4. For toddlers, cut the chicken into strips to serve as finger food with the potato salad, mashed with the back of a fork if needed, and your choice of steamed vegetables.

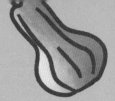

serves **2+4** adults + little ones

prep **15** mins

cook **35** mins

big veg chunky chilli

We've put just enough chilli in this dish to excite + warm tiny taste buds – but if your little one is showing signs of a fiery palate, spice up their life with a teaspoon more!

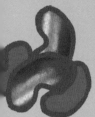

what you need

550 g/1 lb 4 oz **butternut squash**, peeled, deseeded and cut into large bite-sized pieces

1½ tablespoons **olive oil**

1 **onion**, finely chopped

150 g/5½ oz **mushrooms**, roughly chopped

2 large **garlic cloves**, finely chopped

40 g/1½ oz **dried split red lentils**, rinsed

400 ml/14 fl oz **passata** (sieved tomatoes)

400 ml/14 fl oz hot low-salt **vegetable stock**

2 tablespoons **tomato puree**

400 g/14 oz can **red kidney beans** in water, drained and rinsed

5 **cloves**

1 teaspoon **ground ginger**

1 teaspoon **mild chilli powder**

1 teaspoon **dried oregano**

Cooked brown rice, steamed green veg, grated cheese and natural yogurt, to serve

what to do

1. Preheat the oven to 180°C/350°F/Gas Mark 4. Toss the squash in half the oil, then spread it out in a roasting tray and roast in the oven for 25–30 minutes, turning once, until tender and slightly golden.

2. Meanwhile, heat the remaining oil in a large saucepan over a medium heat, add the onion and mushrooms, cover the pan with a lid and cook, stirring frequently, for 6 minutes or until softened.

3. Stir in the garlic and lentils, then add the passata, stock, tomato puree, beans, cloves, ginger, chilli powder and oregano and bring almost to the boil. Reduce the heat, part-cover with a lid and simmer, stirring occasionally, for 25 minutes or until reduced and thickened.

4. When the squash is cooked, stir it into the chilli. Finely chop the chilli for babies, then serve with cooked rice and steamed green veg and topped with grated cheese and a spoonful of yogurt.

just for fun scoop the seeds!

Use an ice-cream scoop to remove the seeds from the squash – it's so quick and easy! And don't forget to save the washed and dried seeds to use in a shaker for your baby.

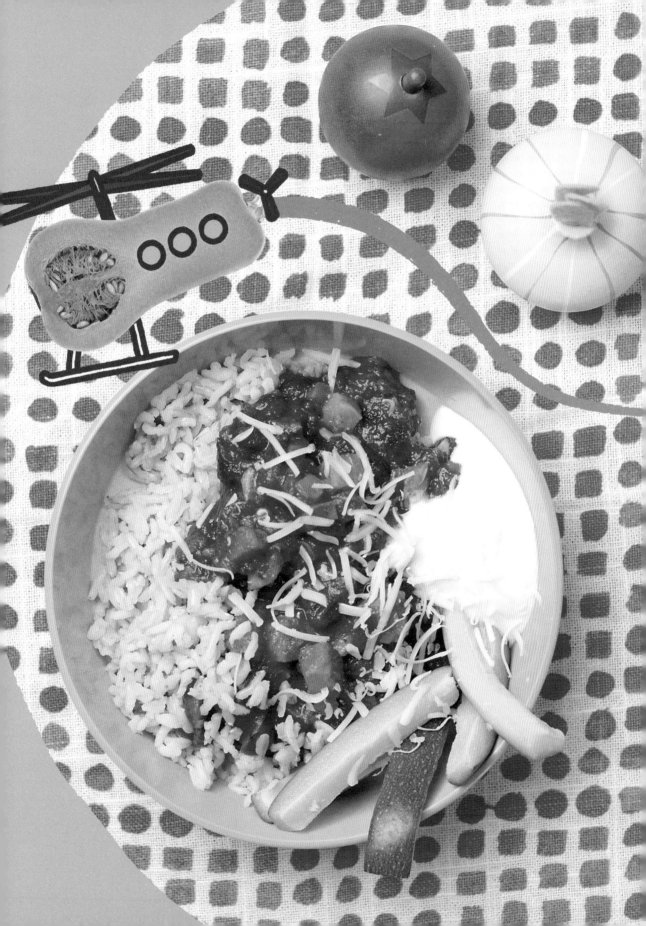

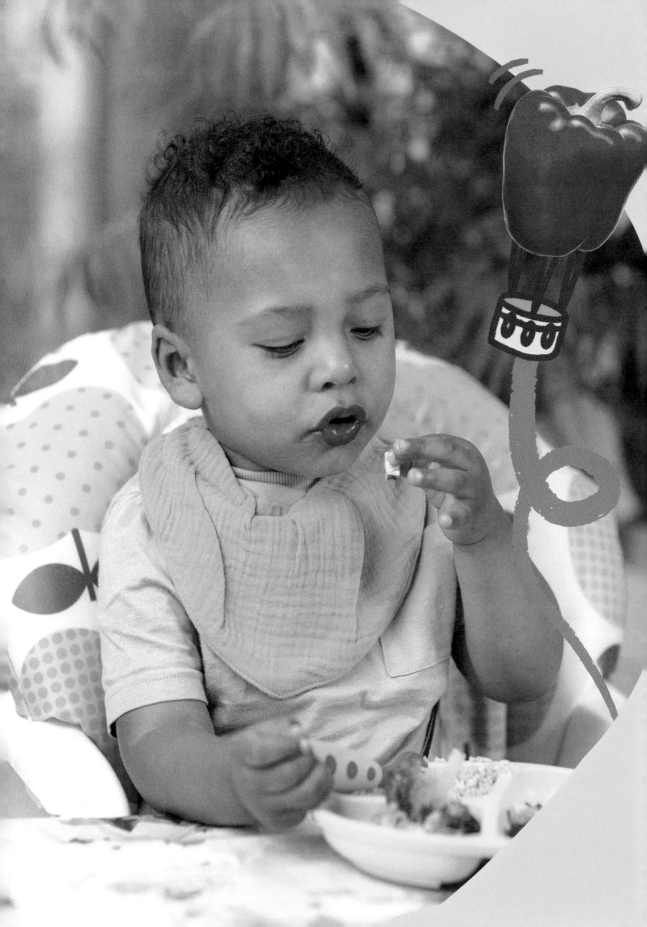

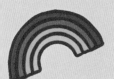

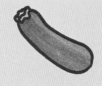

serves 2+2 adults + little ones

prep 20 mins + marinating

cook 15 mins

rainbow veg + tofu kebabs

Eat a rainbow of veggies with these colourful kebabs! The chunks of veg + tofu are great fun for little hands to pick up + for little mouths to explore. Try our suggestions – or mix + match!

what you need

350 g/12 oz firm **smoked or plain tofu**, drained well, patted dry with kitchen paper and cut into 16 cubes

1 small **red pepper**, cored, deseeded and cut into 16 pieces

2 small **courgettes**, sliced into 8 chunks

1 small **yellow pepper**, cored, deseeded and cut into 16 pieces

Olive oil, for drizzling

Toasted sesame seeds, for sprinkling

Cooked brown rice and steamed green veg, to serve

For the marinade

1½ tablespoons reduced-salt **soy sauce**

1 large **garlic clove**, crushed

1 tablespoon **tomato puree**

1½ teaspoons **clear honey**

what to do

1) For the marinade, mix all the ingredients together in a large shallow dish. Add the tofu and turn until coated. Cover and leave to marinate in the fridge for 1 hour, or preferably longer if there is time.

2) Put the vegetables in a bowl and drizzle over a little oil. Toss with your hands to coat.

3) Preheat the grill to high and line a baking sheet with foil. Thread the tofu and vegetables on to 8 skewers in the following order: 1 yellow pepper, 1 tofu, 1 courgette, 1 red pepper, 1 tofu, 1 yellow pepper, 1 red pepper. Place the kebabs on the baking sheet and spoon any leftover marinade over the tofu.

4) Grill the kebabs for 15 minutes, turning halfway through cooking, until the tofu is golden and the veg starts to colour on the edges. Remove the skewers and either chop the tofu and veg into small pieces or serve as finger food. Sprinkle toasted sesame seeds over the tofu and veg and serve with cooked brown rice and steamed green veg. Grown-ups may also like a splash of chilli sauce.

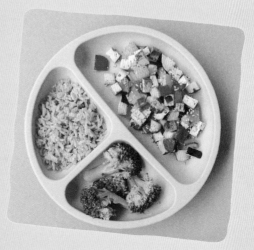

serves
2+2
adults +
little ones

prep
15
mins
+ chilling

cook
40
mins

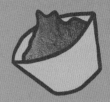

feelin' fine falafel

Chickpeas are a brilliant source of protein.
Let your little one have fun dipping + dunking the
falafel + they'll soon be feelin' fine!

what you need

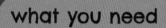

3 **spring onions**, roughly chopped

1 teaspoon **olive oil**, plus extra
  for cooking

400 g/14 oz can **chickpeas** in
  water, drained, plus 1 teaspoon
  water from the can

2 teaspoons **ground coriander**

1 teaspoon **ground cumin**

1 teaspoon **garlic powder**

1/2 teaspoon **baking powder**

3 **sweet potatoes** (about 125 g/
  4 1/2 oz each), scrubbed, halved
  crossways and cut into wedges

To serve

**Cucumber, red pepper and
  avocado**, cut into fingers

**Hummus, mayonnaise or
  Tomato Sauce** (see page 169)

what to do

1. Line a baking sheet with baking parchment.

2. Put the spring onions in a mini food processor
   or blender with the oil and blend until very finely
   chopped. Add the chickpeas and 1 teaspoon of the
   chickpea water and blend again until coarsely
   chopped with some small chunks of chickpea.
   Spoon the mixture into a mixing bowl. Stir the
   spices and baking powder into the chickpea mixture
   to make a thick coarse paste.

3. Divide the chickpea mixture into 10 portions, then
   shape each one into a ball and flatten slightly with
   the palm of your hand. Place on the prepared baking
   sheet and chill for 20 minutes to firm up slightly.

4. Meanwhile, preheat the oven to 200°C/400°F/Gas
   Mark 6. Toss the sweet potato wedges in a little oil,
   then spread out on a separate baking sheet and roast
   for 30–40 minutes, turning halfway.

5. Halfway through cooking the sweet potato wedges,
   brush the tops and sides of the falafel with oil and
   place in the oven. Cook for 20 minutes, turning
   once, until crisp on the outside. Serve the falafel
   with the sweet potato wedges, vegetables fingers
   and your choice of sauce.

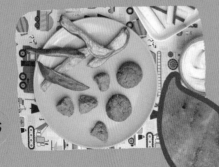

fridge frrrresh!

The cooked falafel will keep in the fridge for up to
3 days and make a quick and easy finger food lunch
with pitta bread, vegetable sticks and a favourite dip.

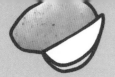

serves
2+2
adults +
little ones

prep
20
mins

cook
30
mins

crispy veggie fingers

Perfect for little hands to feed themselves, these
veggie-packed fingers are crispy + creamy with
a hint of mustard. You can make them from scratch
or use any leftover veggies you have.

veggie-licious!

what you need

325 g/11½ oz **floury potatoes**,
halved

60 g/2¼ oz **white cabbage**,
chopped

90 g/3¼ oz **frozen petits pois**

3 **spring onions**, finely chopped

1 teaspoon **English
mustard powder**

4 tablespoons **cottage cheese**

1 large **egg**, lightly beaten

85 g/3 oz **fresh breadcrumbs**

Sunflower oil, for frying

For the creamy leeks

2 **leeks**, trimmed, cleaned and
thinly sliced

2 tablespoons hot low-salt
vegetable stock

1 tablespoon **cream or
crème fraîche**

what to do

1. Cook the potatoes in a saucepan of boiling water for 12–15 minutes until tender. Drain and leave to dry and cool slightly, then peel off the skins and coarsely grate into a large bowl.

2. Meanwhile, steam or boil the cabbage and petits pois in a saucepan over a medium heat for 3–4 minutes until tender, then finely chop.

3. Add the cabbage and petits pois, spring onions, mustard and cottage cheese to the bowl with the grated potatoes and mix until combined.

4. Place the beaten egg in a shallow bowl and the breadcrumbs on a plate. Divide the potato mixture into 10 equal pieces and shape into fingers. Dip each finger into the beaten egg, then roll in the breadcrumbs until coated all over.

5. Heat enough oil to generously cover the base of a large, nonstick frying pan and cook the veggie fingers in 2 batches over a medium heat for 5–7 minutes, turning occasionally, until golden all over.

6. Meanwhile, make the creamy leeks. Steam the leeks in a saucepan over a medium heat for 4–5 minutes until tender. Transfer them to a mini food processor or blender with the stock and cream and blend until smooth and creamy. Serve with the veggie fingers.

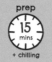

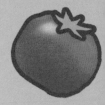
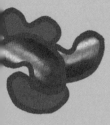

serves **2+2**
adults + little ones

prep **15 mins**
+ chilling

cook **20 mins**

jumpin' bean burgers

Your little one's taste buds will jump for joy when they try these spiced bean burgers – and they are perfect for your freezer stash!

what you need

3 large **spring onions**, roughly chopped

400 g/14 oz can **red kidney beans** in water, drained and rinsed

55 g/2 oz fresh day-old **breadcrumbs**

1 heaped teaspoon **mild smoked paprika**

1 teaspoon **garlic granules**

2 tablespoons **tomato puree**

Plain flour, for dusting

Olive oil, for frying

Warm mini pitta breads or burger buns, split open, **sliced tomato, finely grated carrot and sweet potato wedges** (see page 176), to serve

what to do

1. Put the spring onions and three-quarters of the beans in a food processor and blitz to a coarse puree. Add the remaining beans to the processor and pulse briefly to roughly chop. Spoon the bean mixture into a mixing bowl and stir in the breadcrumbs, paprika, garlic granules and tomato puree and stir until combined.

2. Place enough flour in a shallow bowl to cover the surface and dust your hands with a little extra flour. Divide the bean mixture into 6 equal pieces and shape them into burgers. Dust each burger in the flour until lightly coated all over. Place on a plate and chill for at least 30 minutes to firm up.

3. Heat enough oil to coat the base of a nonstick frying pan over a medium heat and cook the burgers for 3 minutes on each side until golden and warmed through.

4. Place each burger in a warm mini pitta bread or burger bun with slices of tomato and grated carrot. Finely chop or mash the burgers and tomatoes for babies, if necessary. Serve with the sweet potato wedges as finger food on the side.

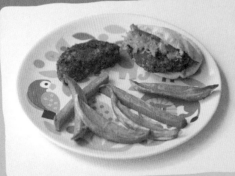

our friends say...

'I make my breadcrumbs using slightly stale leftover bread in batches and then freeze them, ready for when I need them. They're great not only for making homemade burgers, but for fishcakes and breaded chicken strips, too.'

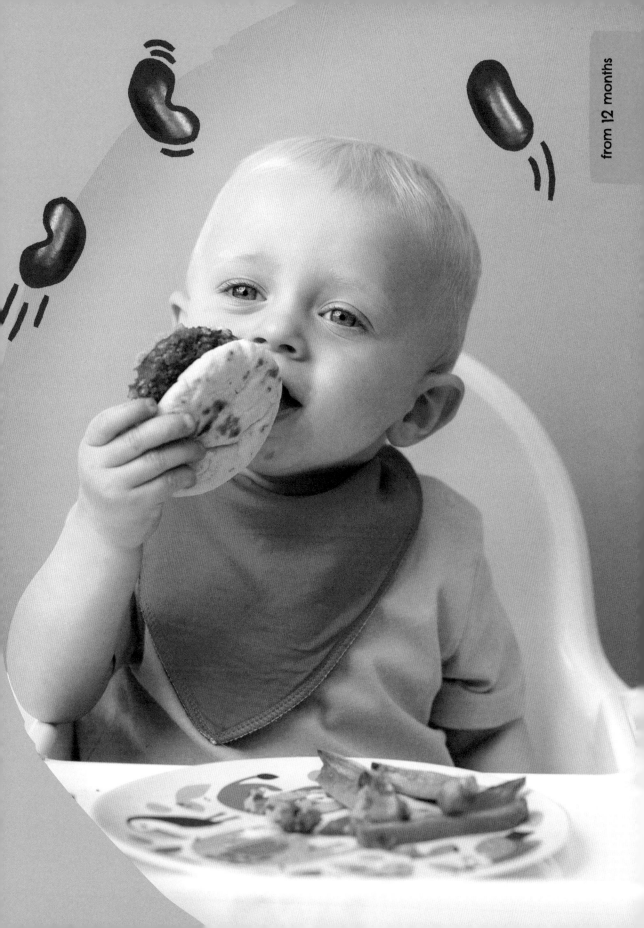

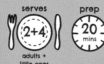

serves **2+4** adults + little ones

prep **20** mins

cook **35** mins

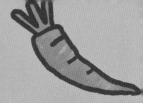
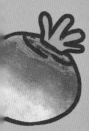

open wide cheesy pie

A family dinner winner, this yummy pie has five different types of tasty veg. Cue big cheesy smiles all round!

what you need

1 tablespoon **olive oil**

60 g/2¼ oz **swede or parsnip**, peeled and diced

2 **carrots**, peeled and diced

2 **leeks**, trimmed, cleaned and thinly sliced

2 large **garlic cloves**, chopped

400 g/14 oz can **chopped tomatoes**

400 g/14 oz can **green lentils** in water, drained and rinsed

1 teaspoon **dried mixed herbs**

550 g/1 lb 4 oz **potatoes**, peeled and cut into large bite-sized pieces

4 tablespoons **whole milk or milk of choice**

1 teaspoon **Dijon mustard**

75 g/2½ oz **Cheddar cheese**, grated

Steamed green veg, to serve

what to do

1) Heat the oil in a large saucepan over a medium–low heat. Add the swede or parsnip, carrots and leeks, part-cover with a lid and cook for 15 minutes, stirring frequently, until softened. Add the garlic, tomatoes, lentils and herbs and cook, part-covered with a lid, for a further 10 minutes or until the vegetables are tender.

2) Meanwhile, cook the potatoes in a large saucepan of boiling water for 12–15 minutes until tender. Drain, then return them to the pan with the milk, mustard and half the cheese. Mash until smooth.

3) Preheat the grill to high. Spoon the vegetable mixture into an ovenproof dish, top with the mash and scatter over the remaining cheese. Grill for 10 minutes or until golden on top. Finely chop the vegetables for babies and serve with steamed green veg.

smelly socks!

Dried herbs are brilliant for sniffing games. Put a teaspoon of dried mint, basil, oregano or mixed herbs in a baby sock (one herb per sock), then let your little one have a good sniff. Play a game matching up the smelly socks to the smells of the herbs in their pots.

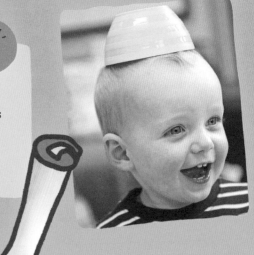

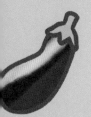

serves **2** prep **10 mins** cook **15 mins**

rat-a-tat-tat-touille

This ratatouille-inspired dish is so delicious it will have your little one saying mmm with every spoon-tapping + lip-licking taste!

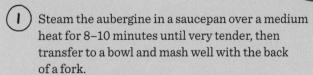

what you need

1 small **aubergine**, peeled and cut into chunks

2 teaspoons **olive oil**

4 tablespoons drained **canned chickpeas** in water, rinsed

1 **garlic clove**, crushed

200 ml/7 fl oz **passata** (sieved tomatoes)

1/2 teaspoon **dried oregano**

1/2 teaspoon **mild smoked paprika**

50 g/1³/4 oz **frozen chopped spinach**

2 tablespoons **cooked couscous**

2 teaspoons **hummus** (optional) and **steamed fine green beans**, to serve

what to do

1. Steam the aubergine in a saucepan over a medium heat for 8–10 minutes until very tender, then transfer to a bowl and mash well with the back of a fork.

2. Meanwhile, heat the oil in a small saucepan over a medium–low heat and add the chickpeas and garlic and cook, stirring, for 1 minute. Add the passata, oregano, paprika and 3 tablespoons of water and simmer, part-covered and stirring occasionally, for 5 minutes.

3. Add the cooked aubergine and spinach and cook for another 5 minutes or until heated through. Blend with a hand blender or mash with the back of fork, making sure the chickpeas are broken down to a coarse puree, adding a splash of hot water if needed.

4. Stir in the cooked couscous. Serve in bowls with a spoonful of hummus stirred in (if using) and green beans on the side as finger food.

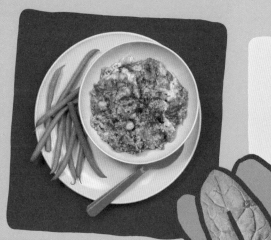

full of beans!

Swap the chickpeas for any canned white beans you have in the cupboard. Feel free to change the spinach for any finely chopped leafy green veg, too.

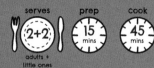

serves 2+2 adults + little ones | prep 15 mins | cook 45 mins

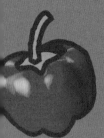

little fishy in a dishy

This exciting fishy dishy combines warming spices –
turmeric + ras el hanout – with chunky white fish.

what you need

1 1/2 teaspoons **ras el hanout spice mix**

1 teaspoon **ground turmeric**

375 g/13 oz thick skinless **white fish fillets**, patted dry, cut into 2.5 cm/1 inch chunks

1 tablespoon **olive oil**

1 **onion**, finely chopped

1 **red pepper**, cored, deseeded and finely chopped

2 **garlic cloves**, finely chopped

50 g/1 3/4 oz **dried red split lentils**, rinsed

400 ml/14 fl oz hot low-salt **vegetable stock**

400 g/14 oz can **chopped tomatoes**

75 g/2 1/2 oz **frozen chopped spinach**, defrosted

Natural Greek yogurt and cooked couscous, to serve

what to do

1. Mix together half of the ras el hanout and the turmeric in a shallow dish. Add the fish and turn to coat. Cover and set aside in the fridge until needed.

2. Heat the oil in a saucepan over a medium–low heat, add the onion and pepper, stir and cover with a lid. Cook the vegetables, stirring occasionally, for 10 minutes or until very soft. Stir in the garlic, lentils and the remaining ras el hanout spice mix, then pour in the stock and chopped tomatoes.

3. Turn the heat up to medium and when the stock starts to bubble, reduce the heat and simmer for 20–25 minutes, part-covered with the lid and stirring occasionally. When the lentils are tender, stir in the spinach and add the fish, gently stirring to cover it in the sauce. Cook over a low heat for 5–8 minutes until the fish is cooked through.

4. Spoon into bowls and break up any large pieces of fish with the back of a fork. Serve with a spoonful of yogurt on top and cooked couscous – stir both into the sauce if serving to little ones.

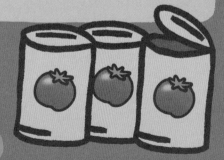

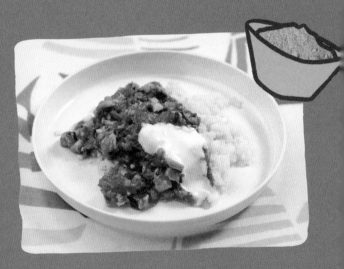

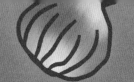

serves
2+3
adults +
little ones

prep
15 mins

cook
25 mins

plate-me-up prawn + tomato orzo

This easy one-pan meal is ideal for the whole fam! Packed with juicy prawns, herbs + spices, it will take little mouths on a tasty adventure.

what you need

1 tablespoon **olive oil**

1 **onion**, finely chopped

1 **red pepper**, cored, deseeded and finely chopped

2 **celery sticks**, finely chopped

2 **garlic cloves**, crushed

2 teaspoons **Cajun spice mix or mild smoked paprika**

1 teaspoon **dried oregano**

200 g/7oz **dried orzo pasta**

500 ml/18 fl oz **passata** (sieved tomatoes)

500 ml/18 fl oz hot low-salt **chicken or vegetable stock**

200 g/7 oz **small frozen prawns**, defrosted

Squeeze of **lemon juice**

100 g/3½ oz **feta cheese**, crumbled (optional)

Steamed green veg, to serve

what to do

1. Heat the oil in a deep sauté pan over a medium–low heat. Add the onion, red pepper and celery and cook, covered with a lid and stirring occasionally, for 8–10 minutes until softened. Stir in the garlic, spices and oregano.

2. Add the orzo, passata and stock, mix until combined, then spread out evenly in the pan and bring to a gentle bubble. Cook, stirring occasionally to prevent the pasta sticking to the bottom of the pan, for 8 minutes or until the pasta is almost tender. Stir in the prawns, add a good squeeze of lemon juice and cook for 2–3 minutes until the pasta is cooked and the prawns have heated through.

3. Spoon into bowls, cutting up the pasta and prawns for your toddler, if needed. Scatter feta over the top or stir it in (if using) and serve with steamed green veg.

super swaps!

Swap the prawns for cooked chicken or pork, cubes of tofu, canned beans or fillets of fish.

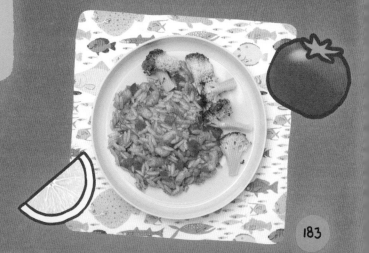

183

serves **2+2** adults + little ones

 prep **15** mins

 cook **25** mins

slam dunk satay chicken

Just right for little tums, the juicy strips of chicken
with the golden peanutty sauce are so deeelicious,
they're a slam dunk!

what you need

3 skinless **chicken breasts**

5 cm/2 inch piece of **fresh root ginger**, peeled and sliced

2 large **garlic cloves**, peeled and halved

1 tablespoon reduced-salt **soy sauce**

3 **spring onions**, finely chopped

200 g/7 oz small **broccoli florets**

Handful of **sugar snap peas**

700 g/1 lb 9 oz **cooked thick udon noodles**

For the satay sauce

3 tablespoons no-salt, no-sugar **smooth peanut butter**

1/2 teaspoon reduced-salt **soy sauce**

2 tablespoons **coconut milk or mayonnaise**

what to do

1. Put the chicken breasts in a deep sauté pan with a lid. Add the ginger, garlic and soy sauce. Pour in enough just-boiled water to just cover the chicken. Put the lid on and simmer gently for 15–20 minutes until the chicken is cooked through and there is no sign of pink in the middle – don't let the chicken overcook or it will be dry.

2. Meanwhile, make the satay sauce. Mix all the ingredients together in a bowl and set aside.

3. Using a slotted spoon, remove the chicken, garlic and ginger from the broth. Cover the chicken to keep it warm and set aside. Discard the garlic and ginger.

4. Add the spring onions, broccoli and sugar snap peas to the hot broth and cook for 1 minute, then add the noodles and heat through for 2 minutes, stirring gently with a fork to loosen them into individual strands.

5. Using a slotted spoon, remove the noodles and veg from the broth and chop into 1 cm/1/2 inch pieces. Finely shred the chicken. Divide the noodles, veg and chicken among bowls and add a spoonful of broth and satay sauce before stirring well. To serve finger food style, chop the noodles, cut the chicken and veg into fingers and serve on a plate, with a small bowl of satay sauce for dunking.

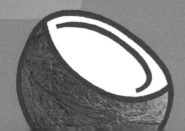

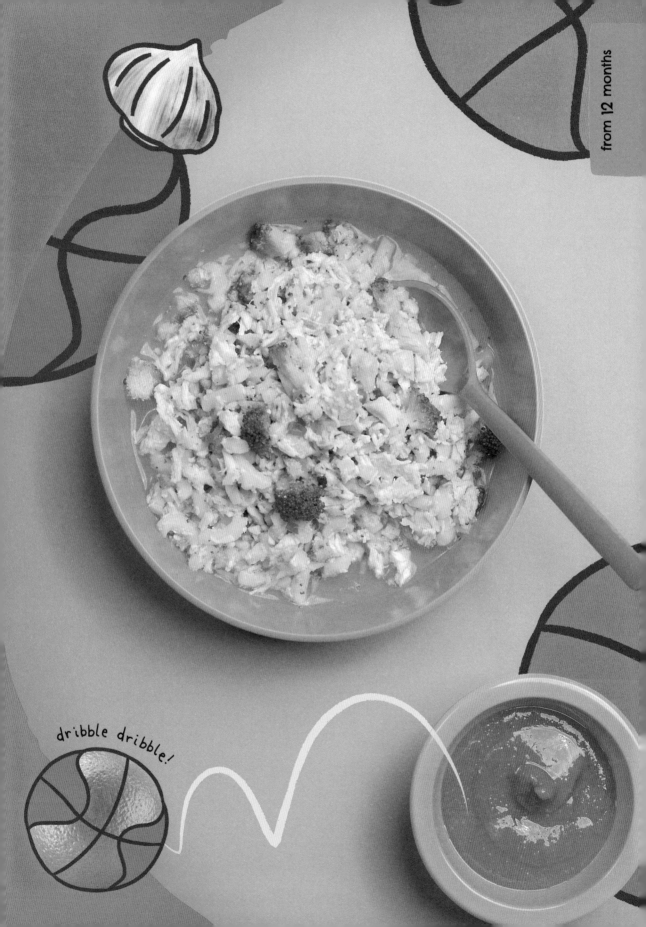

from 12 months

dribble dribble!

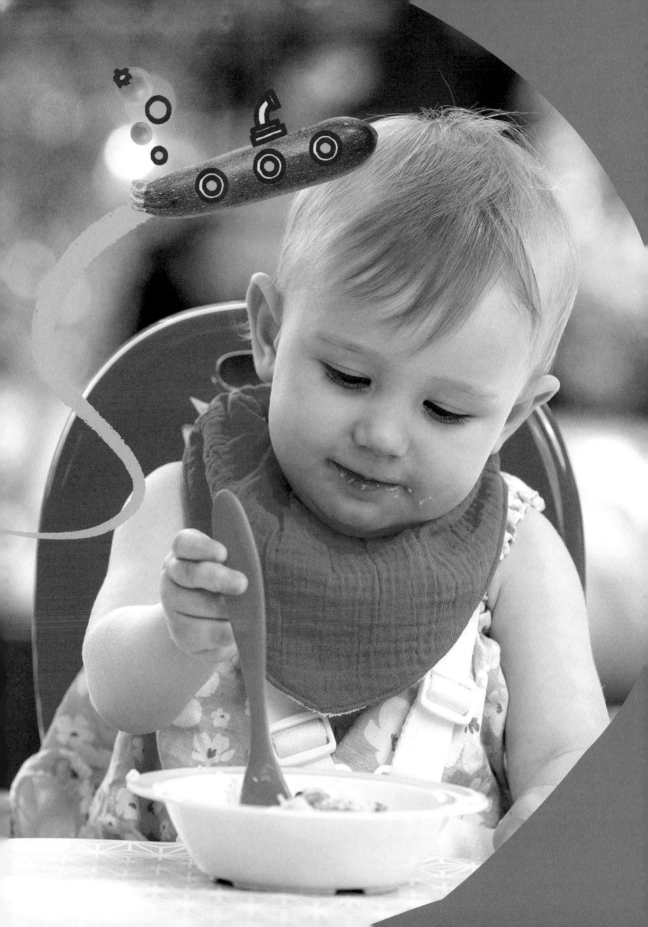

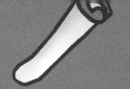

serves **2+2** adults + little ones

prep **15** mins

cook **20** mins

squish-squish dinky dumplings

This recipe uses ready-made gnocchi as the perfect cheat for squishy dumplings. Served with a creamy, veggie-packed sauce, these dinky dumplings are just pea-fect!

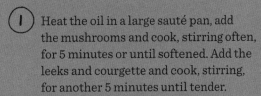

what you need

1 tablespoon **olive oil**

200 g/7 oz **mushrooms**, finely chopped

2 **leeks**, trimmed, cleaned and finely chopped

1 **courgette**, diced

300 ml/$\frac{1}{2}$ pint hot low-salt **vegetable stock**

400 ml/14 fl oz **whole milk or milk of choice**

$1\frac{1}{2}$ tablespoons **cornflour**

1 teaspoon **English mustard**

60 g/$2\frac{1}{4}$ oz **mature Cheddar cheese**, grated

100 g/$3\frac{1}{2}$ oz **frozen peas**

400 g/14 oz **gnocchi**

Freshly ground **black pepper**

what to do

1. Heat the oil in a large sauté pan, add the mushrooms and cook, stirring often, for 5 minutes or until softened. Add the leeks and courgette and cook, stirring, for another 5 minutes until tender.

2. Pour the stock into the pan. Mix 2 tablespoons of the milk into the cornflour in a small bowl, then add to the pan with the remaining milk. Bring almost to the boil, then turn the heat down and simmer for 10 minutes or until thickened to a smooth, creamy sauce. Stir in the mustard and cheese, then season with pepper.

3. Meanwhile, bring a large saucepan of water to the boil. Add the peas and gnocchi, return to the boil and cook for 4–5 minutes until tender – the gnocchi will rise to the surface when it is ready. Drain the gnocchi and peas, reserving some of the cooking water.

4. Add the gnocchi and peas to the pan with the creamy sauce. Stir until everything is combined, adding a spoonful of the reserved cooking water if needed. Spoon into bowls and cut the gnocchi up for your toddler, if needed.

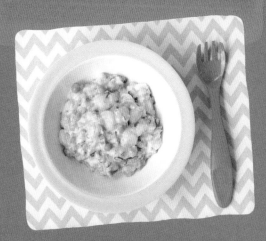

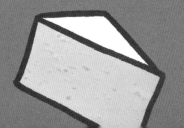

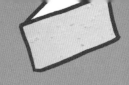

serves **2+2** adults + little ones | prep **15** mins | cook **40** mins

tuck-in turkey + fennel pasta bake

This yummy pasta bake, which offers the new + exciting flavour of fennel, is perfect for stretching tiny taste buds! It's so good that the whole family will gobble it up!

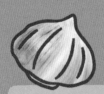

what you need

1 tablespoon **olive oil**

400 g/14 oz skinless **turkey breast**, cut into bite-sized pieces

2 **garlic cloves**, finely chopped

1 teaspoon **dried oregano**

1/2 teaspoon **fennel seeds**

400 g/14 oz can **chopped tomatoes**

1 tablespoon **tomato puree**

280 g/10 oz **dried penne pasta**

125 g/41/2 oz **mozzarella cheese**, torn into pieces

Steamed green veg of choice, to serve

what to do

1. Preheat the oven to 190°C/375°F/Gas Mark 5. Heat the oil in a nonstick frying pan over a medium–high heat, add the turkey and cook, turning occasionally, for 5 minutes or until browned. Remove with a slotted spoon and set aside.

2. Reduce the heat to medium–low, add the garlic, oregano and fennel seeds to the pan and stir, then add the tomatoes and tomato puree. Bring to the boil, then reduce the heat, part-cover with a lid and simmer, stirring frequently, for 10 minutes or until reduced and thickened.

3. Meanwhile, cook the pasta in a saucepan of boiling water for about 1 minute less than the packet instructions or until just tender. Drain, reserving the cooking water.

4. Return the pasta and 100 ml/31/2 fl oz of the reserved cooking water to the saucepan, stir in the turkey and the tomato sauce and warm through. Tip the pasta mixture into an ovenproof dish and scatter the mozzarella over the top.

5. Cover the pasta with a lid or foil and bake in the oven for 10 minutes, then remove the lid or foil and cook for a further 10 minutes or until the mozzarella has melted and the turkey is cooked through. Finely chop the pasta bake for babies before serving with steamed green veg of your choice.

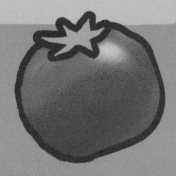
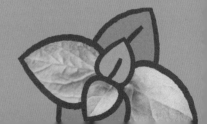

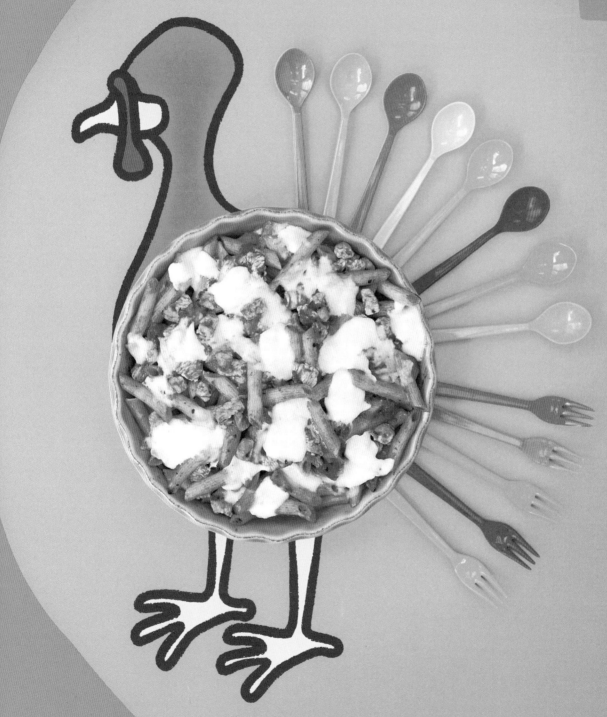

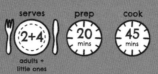

serves
2+4
adults +
little ones

prep
20 mins

cook
45 mins

chicken paella-ella-ella

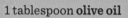

Taste a rainbow of yummy veggies, including tomatoes
+ peas, with this one-pot wonder. Veggie-licious!

what you need

1 tablespoon **olive oil**

2 **unsmoked bacon rashers**, cut into small pieces

4 skinless, boneless **chicken thighs** (about 400 g/14 oz), cut into bite-sized pieces

1 **onion**, finely chopped

1 small **red pepper**, cored, deseeded and chopped

2 **garlic cloves**, finely chopped

225 g/8 oz **paella rice**

Large pinch of **saffron threads** or 1 teaspoon **ground turmeric**

1 heaped teaspoon **mild smoked paprika**

1 teaspoon **dried thyme**

725 ml/26 fl oz low-salt hot **chicken stock**

100 g/3½ oz **frozen petits pois**

4 **tomatoes**, deseeded and diced

Juice of ½ **lemon**

what to do

1. Heat the oil in a large, nonstick frying pan over a medium heat and cook the bacon for 5 minutes or until almost crisp. Remove with a slotted spoon and set aside. Add the chicken to the pan, in 2 batches, and cook each batch for 5 minutes or until the chicken is browned all over. Remove with the slotted spoon and set aside.

2. Reduce the heat slightly, add the onion and red pepper to the pan and cook, stirring frequently, for 5 minutes or until softened. Add the garlic and rice and return the bacon and chicken to the pan. Stir until combined.

3. Mix the saffron or turmeric, paprika and thyme into the hot stock and pour it into the pan. Bring to the boil, then reduce the heat and simmer for 15 minutes, without stirring. Add the petits pois and tomatoes, press them into the rice and cook for a further 10 minutes or until the chicken is cooked through and the rice is tender. Pour over the lemon juice, cover and leave to stand for 5 minutes. Finely chop the paella for babies before serving.

just for fun
have a carnival!

Eating together is the perfect reason to celebrate – turn teatime into a family festival. Find whistles and blowers and make some noise! Make sure everyone has a party hat, too!

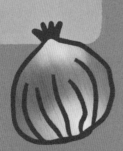

serves **2+3** adults + little ones | prep **15** mins | cook **30** mins

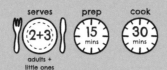

quick + easy cheesy lasagne

Made in one pan, this easy, speedy recipe has all the flavour of a classic lasagne but is ready in half the time. Pasta la vista, baby!

what you need

1 tablespoon **olive oil**

400 g/14 oz **minced beef**, finely chopped

1 large **onion**, diced

1 large **carrot** (about 125 g/4½ oz), coarsely grated

1 large **celery stick**, finely chopped

2 **garlic cloves**, finely chopped

2 teaspoons **dried oregano**

600 g/1 lb 5 oz **canned chopped tomatoes**

300 ml/½ pint low-salt **beef stock**

3 tablespoons **whole milk or milk of choice**

5 sheets of **fresh lasagne**, about 225 g/8 oz total weight, cut into 1 cm/½ inch pieces

5 tablespoons **ricotta cheese**

3 tablespoons finely grated **Parmesan cheese**

Freshly ground **black pepper**

Steamed green veg, to serve (optional)

what to do

1. Heat the oil in a large, deep frying pan over a medium–high heat. Add the minced beef, onion, carrot and celery and cook, stirring to break up any clumps of meat, for 12–15 minutes or until the mince is browned all over and the vegetables have softened.

2. Add the garlic, oregano, tomatoes and stock and cook over a medium heat. When the sauce starts to bubble, turn the heat down to low and simmer, covered with a lid, for 5 minutes or until reduced slightly. Stir in the milk.

3. Season with a little pepper and add the chopped lasagne sheets to the pan, mixing them in evenly. Cover with a lid and cook for 10 minutes until the lasagne is tender.

4. Spoon the ricotta on top of the lasagne and serve sprinkled with Parmesan, with green veg on the side, if liked.

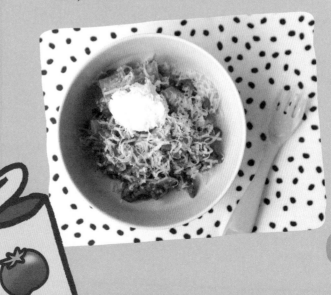

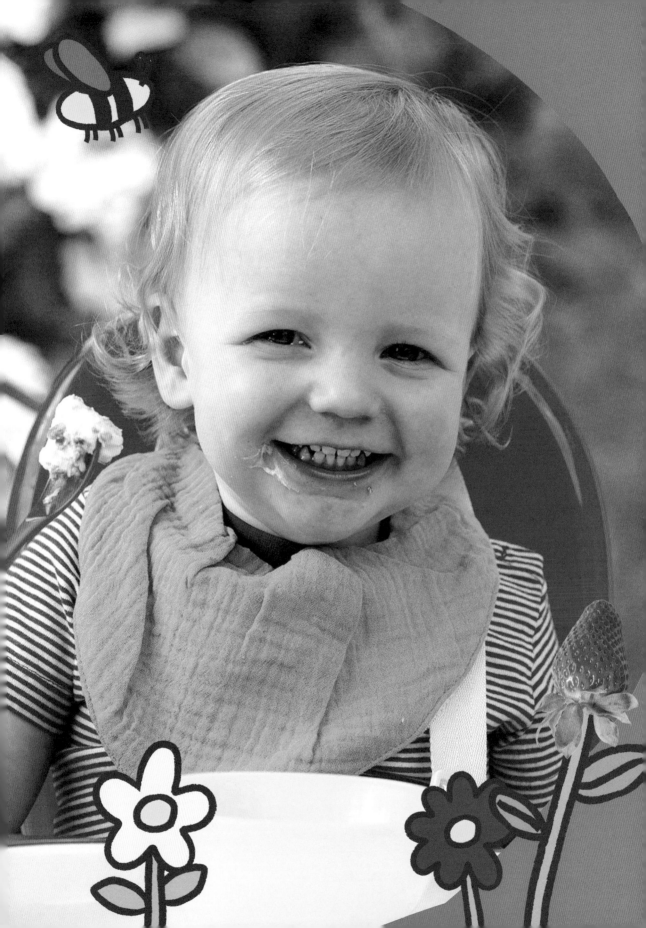

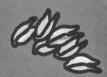

 serves **4**

 prep **10** mins
+ cooling

 cook **10** mins

berry-licious yogurt pots

There are three layers of yumminess in this perfect pudding: a fruity bottom, a creeeamy middle + a crunchy top! Let your little one help to build their own so they can practise their super spoon skills.

what you need

20 g/¾ oz **pecan nuts**

1 tablespoon **sunflower seeds**

3 tablespoons **porridge oats**

2 teaspoons **clear honey**

250 g/9 oz **strawberries or your favourite berries**, hulled

1 teaspoon **vanilla extract**

250 ml/9 fl oz **natural Greek yogurt**

what to do

1) Place the pecans and sunflower seeds in a large, nonstick frying pan over a medium–low heat and dry-fry, turning occasionally, for 3–4 minutes until slightly browned. Keep an eye on them, as they can easily burn. Remove from the pan and finely chop, then tip into a bowl and leave to cool.

2) Add the oats to the pan and dry-fry over a medium–low heat, turning occasionally, for 3–4 minutes until toasted and slightly browned. Tip into the bowl with the pecans and leave to cool. Stir in the honey until everything is coated.

3) Puree 50 g/1¾ oz of the berries in a food processor, or using a hand blender, then stir in the vanilla. Finely chop the remaining berries and stir them into the puree. Divide the berry mixture equally between 4 bowls. Top with yogurt and then the oat mixture just before serving. (You may have some of the oat mixture left over; it will keep, stored in an airtight container, for up to 3 days.)

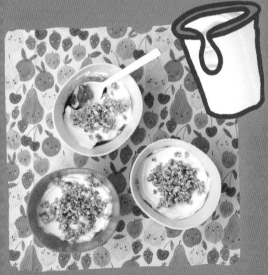

Ella's shortcut!

You can use any of your favourite Ella's Kitchen fruit pouches to make these puds – we love apples, apples, apples or pears, pears, pears or bananas, bananas, bananas!

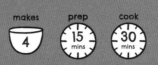

makes 4 · prep 15 mins · cook 30 mins

all-for-me apple crumbles

Suuuuper simple but totally tasty, we love these individual crumbles. Halve the apples, top with crumble mix + bake. Apple-solutely delicious!

what you need

2 **eating apples**, halved horizontally

For the crumble mix

40 g/1½ oz **plain flour**

30 g/1 oz chilled **unsalted butter**, cubed, plus extra for greasing

1 ripe **banana**, finely chopped

1 teaspoon **ground cinnamon**

1 tablespoon **ground mixed seeds**

2 tablespoons **porridge oats**

what to do

1. Preheat the oven to 190°C/375°F/Gas Mark 5. To make the crumble mix, place the flour in a bowl, add the butter and rub in with your fingertips until the mixture resembles coarse breadcrumbs. Stir in the banana, cinnamon, ground seeds and oats.

2. Using a teaspoon, scoop out the core from each apple half. Rub a little butter over the top of each half and sprinkle the crumble mixture over. Place the apples in a small roasting tin, packing them tightly together, and add 1 tablespoon of water to the tin. Bake in the oven for 25–30 minutes until the apples are tender and the crumble is crisp.

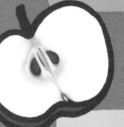

can I help?

When you're little, what could be better than squishing together butter and flour? Let your little one have a go at making crumble. Oooh...messy fingers!

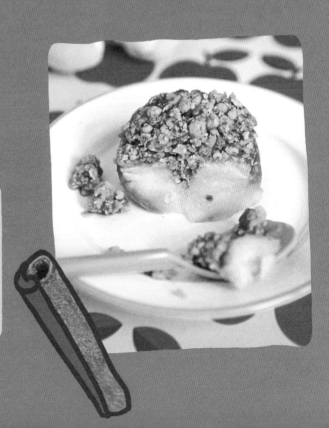

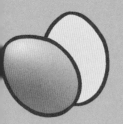

makes
16

prep
20 mins

cook
20 mins

perfect little puffs

For a quick grab + go finger food, try these easy-peasy little puffs. Don't forget to make a few extras for grown-ups to nibble on, too!

what you need

Unsalted butter, for greasing

1 large ripe **banana**

2 tablespoons **ricotta cheese**

320 g/11¼ oz ready-rolled **puff pastry**

Plain flour, for dusting

Beaten egg, to glaze

what to do

1. Preheat the oven to 200°C/400°F/Gas Mark 6. Lightly grease 2 baking sheets.

2. Using the back of a fork, roughly mash the banana in a bowl, then stir in the ricotta.

3. Lay the pastry on a lightly floured work surface and roll it out slightly. Stamp out 32 rounds using a 5 cm/2 inch fluted cutter (re-rolling the trimmings as necessary). Place a heaped teaspoon of banana mixture in the centre of one pastry round and brush the edge with beaten egg. Place a second pastry round on top and gently press the edges together to seal. Place the parcel on a prepared baking sheet. Repeat with the remaining pastry rounds and filling to make 16 parcels.

4. Lightly brush the top of each parcel with beaten egg and prick once with a fork. Bake in the oven for 18–20 minutes until risen and golden. Transfer to a wire rack to cool slightly. Serve warm or cold.

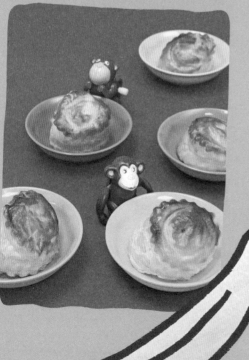

can I help?

With a little bit of grown-up help, your baby can have a go at rolling the pastry and pressing out the rounds. Have fun squidging the leftover pastry pieces, too.

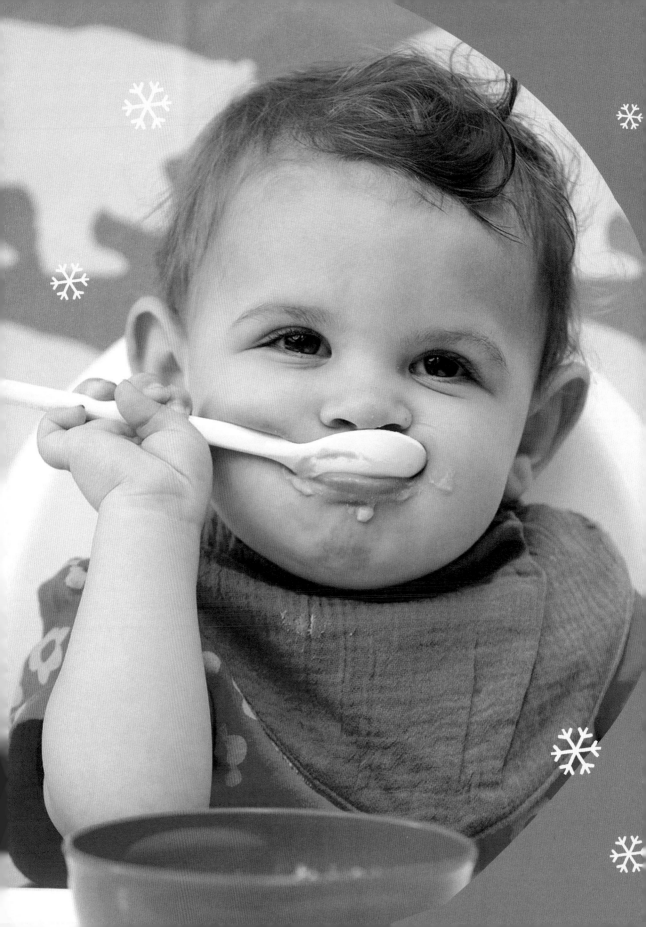

serves
2

prep
5 mins
+ freezing

cook
no cook

cool-me-down banana + peanut ice cream

This brrrilliant ice cream is a cool, healthy alternative to shop-bought ice cream, and with yummy fresh banana + peanut butter, it tastes better too!

what you need

2 large ripe **bananas**, peeled

1 tablespoon no-salt, no-sugar smooth or crunchy **peanut butter**

2 tablespoons **double cream**

what to do

1. Put the bananas in a freezer bag, seal and place in the freezer until frozen.

2. Remove the bananas from the freezer when firm and allow to soften slightly for 10–15 minutes. Break the bananas into pieces and place in a mini food processor or blender with the peanut butter and cream and pulse until smooth and creamy. Spoon into bowls and serve.

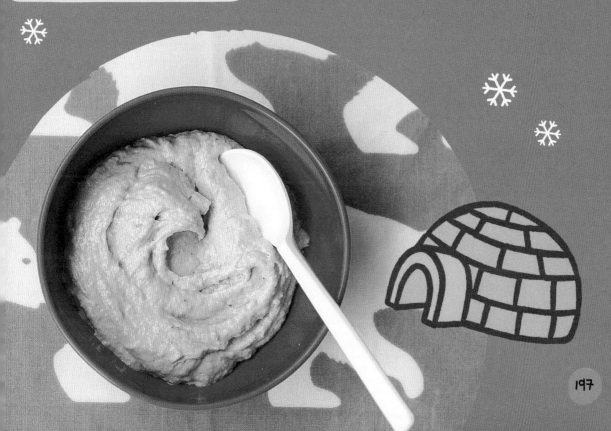

197

serves **5**

prep **10** mins

cook **30** mins

+ resting/cooling

cheeky cherry custard pud

This cheeky pud will have you coming back for more!
Perfect for a little treat, + using frozen fruit for ease,
it's cherrific!

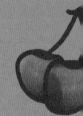

what you need

85 g/3 oz **frozen dark pitted cherries** (about 15), defrosted

10 g/¼ oz **unsalted butter**, plus extra for greasing

2 **eggs**

30 g/1 oz **plain flour**

1 teaspoon **vanilla extract**

1¾ tablespoons **caster sugar**

125 ml/4 fl oz **whole milk or milk of choice**

Freshly grated **nutmeg**, to serve (optional)

what to do

1. Drain and pat dry the defrosted cherries with kitchen paper. Cut the cherries into small pieces.

2. Melt the butter in a small saucepan and leave to cool. Grease a small oven dish with extra butter and arrange the cherries over the base.

3. Put the cooled melted butter, eggs, flour, vanilla, sugar and milk in a mini food processor or blender and pulse for 1–2 minutes to make a smooth batter. Leave to rest for 15 minutes or until ready to bake.

4. Meanwhile, preheat the oven to 180°C/350°F/ Gas Mark 4. Pour the custard into the oven dish over the cherries and place it in a baking tin. Pour enough just-boiled water into the tin to come two-thirds of the way up the sides of oven dish, then carefully put the tin in the oven. Bake for 25–30 minutes or until the custard has just set.

5. Remove the oven dish from the tin and leave for 10 minutes to cool down slightly or until ready to eat. Finely grate a little nutmeg over the custard (if using). The custard can also be served cold and will keep in the fridge for 2 days.

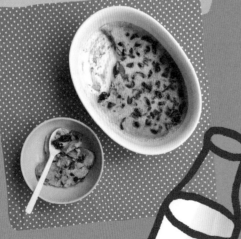

super swaps!

Swap the cherries for blueberries or other berries, chopped nectarines or plums.

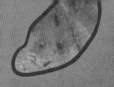

serves **2**   prep **10** mins   cook no cook

oh-so-fruity yogurt pots

Life's a peach with these fruity yogurt pots, which are easy to prep in advance. Keep them chilling in the fridge for a healthy treat.

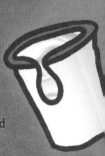

what to do

① Cut the sweet potato in half and scoop out the flesh into a food processor or blender. Add three-quarters of the nectarines or peaches, and the mixed spice, and blend to a puree.

② In a bowl, beat together the yogurt, honey and tahini (if using) until combined.

③ Spoon the yogurt mixture into 2 beakers or bowls, layering it with the puree, and serve topped with the remaining fruit or chill until ready to eat.

what you need

1 small cooked and cooled **sweet potato** (about 100 g/3¹/₂ oz)

2 ripe **nectarines or peaches**, halved, stoned and roughly chopped

¹/₄ teaspoon **ground mixed spice**

150 ml/5¹/₂ fl oz **natural Greek yogurt**

1 teaspoon **clear honey**

1 tablespoon **tahini** (optional)

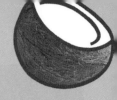

best-of-the-bunch banana muffins

makes 12 **prep** 10 mins + cooling **cook** 15 mins

30 g/1 oz **unsalted butter**, melted, plus extra for greasing

1 ripe **banana**, peeled and cut into quarters

2 tablespoons **maple syrup or clear honey**

1 **egg**

60 g/2¼ oz **self-raising flour**

¼ teaspoon **ground cinnamon**

2 teaspoons **ground mixed seeds**

Fresh fruit, such as strawberries, halved or quartered, depending on size, to serve (optional)

Preheat the oven to 180°C/350°F/Gas Mark 4. Grease 12 holes of a mini-muffin tin with butter.

Put the banana in a mini food processor or blender and pulse until almost smooth. Add the remaining ingredients and blend until just combined.

Divide the muffin mixture evenly between the holes and bake in the oven for 12–15 minutes until risen and cooked through. Leave in the tin for 5 minutes, then turn out on to a wire rack to cool completely. Serve on their own or with fresh fruit on the side (if using).

mango-nificent coconut rice pud

serves 2–4 **prep** 5 mins **cook** 30 mins

100 g/3½ oz **risotto rice**

450 ml/16 fl oz **unsweetened coconut drinking milk**

½ teaspoon **vanilla extract**

½ teaspoon **ground cinnamon**

1½ tablespoons **clear honey or maple syrup**

75 g/2½ oz ripe **mango**, diced

Tip the rice into a saucepan and pour in the coconut drinking milk. Heat over a medium–low heat until the milk starts to bubble, then stir in the vanilla, cinnamon and honey or maple syrup.

Turn the heat to low, cover with a lid and simmer, stirring regularly, for 25 minutes or until the rice is tender. Serve warm or cold topped with the mango.

super swaps!

Swap the mango for your little one's favourite fruit – banana, cooked apple or pear, nectarine, peach or pineapple are all yum.

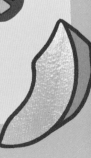

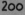

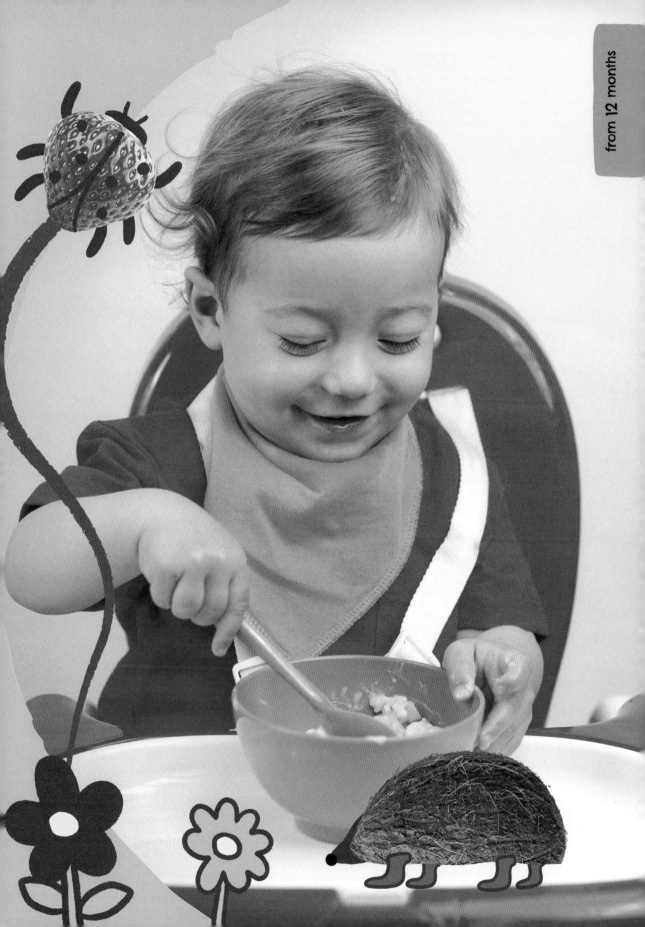

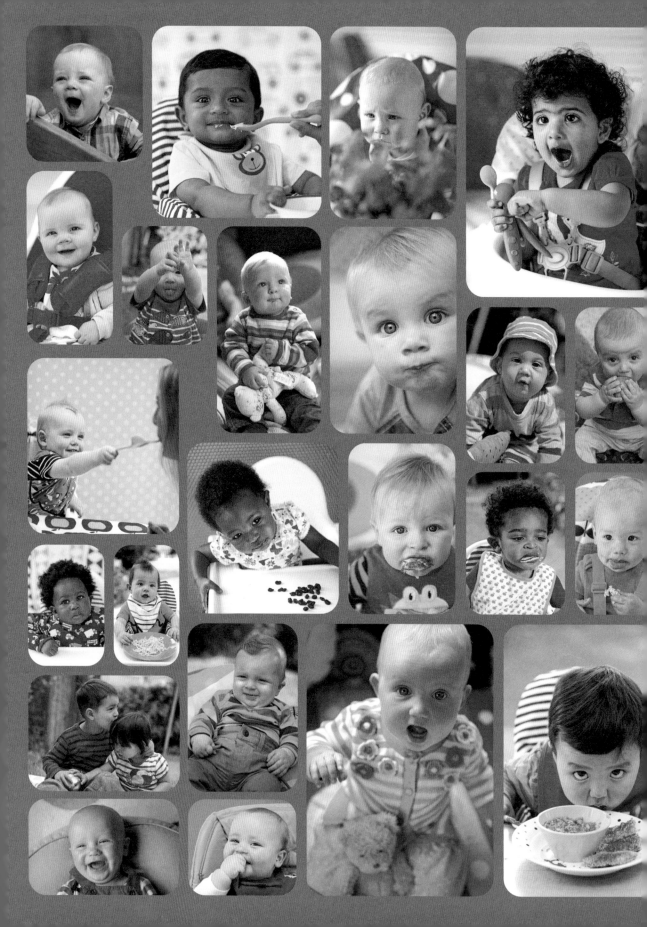

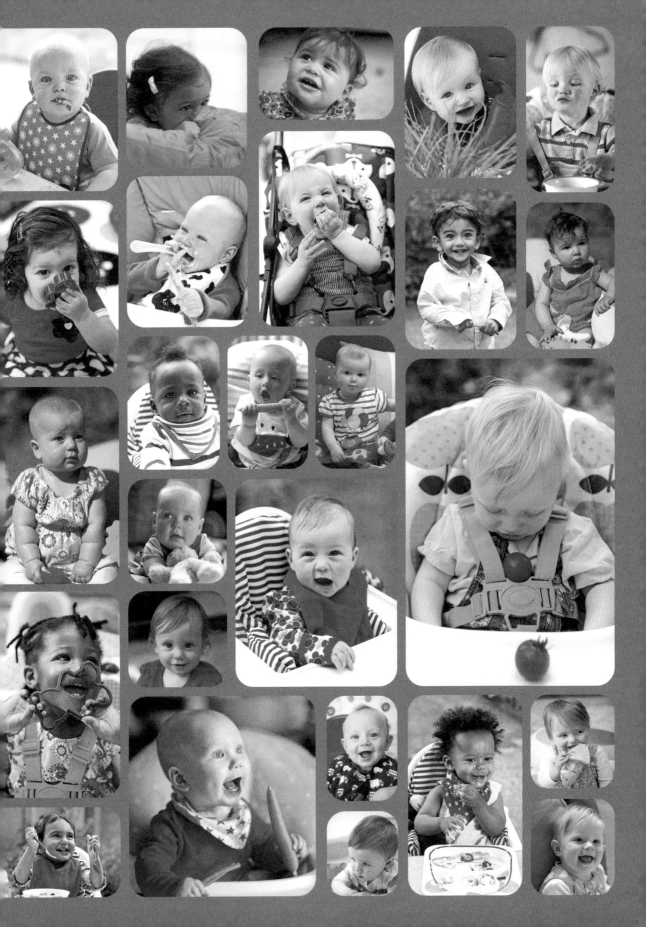

UK/US terms

index

thank you

A big thank you to all of the Ella's Kitchen employees + friends who contributed recipe ideas for this book + 'road-tested' them with their own families.

A huge thank you to Brother Max, Cosatto, JoJo Maman Bébé, Marimekko, Next, Rice, Skibz + Tomy for their kind supply of colourful clothes + equipment, which helped make our photographs all the more lovely.

A special thank you to all our little helpers – and their parents + carers – who have appeared in the various editions of *Ella's Kitchen First Foods* over the years. Here's a list of our little stars + their ages on the days of our photoshoots.

Aaruhi Pindoria (14 months) • Adam Brefo (11 months) • Adriana Bussandri Morais (11 months) • Alex Schembri (3 years) • Alfie Symons (10 months) • Amilia Rose Morrison (17 months) • Amy Powell (6 months) • Anima Tavares (11 months) • Astrid O'Connor (13 months) • Austin Van de Peer (12 months) • Ava Crick (20 months) • Benjamin Lee (7 months) • Bertie Ball (13 months) • Betsy Swaffer (10 months) • Bruce Burton (7 months) • Carter-Jay Moka (2 years) • Charlie Nichols (11 months) • Cleo Stokes-McDonnell (20 months) • Creedan-Lee Moka (6 months) • Delphine Wetz (6 months) • Dilan Johal (12 months) • Edie Carter (14 months) • Elohor Oghoyone (6 months) • Eloise Mills (6 months) • Eloise-Rose Ludlow-Wade (11 months) • Emilia Dames (8 months) • Emilia Kooyman (6 months) • Esha Patel (10 months) • Esther Sax-Lewis (8 months) • Evelyn Bolton (7 months) • Ezra Sax-Lewis (8 months) • Ezra Vincent-Little (20 months) • Finn Jennings (17 months) • Florence Pallent (7 months) • Freya Champaneri (18 months) • Freya Phoenix Kelly (10 months) • Harriet King (9 months) • Harrison McDonnell (7 months) • Harry Belmore (10 months) • Holly Crawford (10 months) • Hugo Tang (7 months) • IreOluwa Ade-Onojobi (7 months) • Jack Jensen-Humphreys (17 months) • Jai-Han Marshall (11 months) • Jasmine Layla Bryan (13 months) • Jessica Laycock (9 months) • Joseph Bartlett (6 months) • Joseph Cartlidge (7 months) • Joshua Davis (7 months) • Katharine English (8 months) • Koa De Guzman (12 months) • Lilah Lewis (13 months) • Luther Morgan (8 months) • Maeva Moon (8 months) • Matilda Friend (8 months) • Matilda Schembri (11 months) • Max McGinty (14 months)

• Mia Joelle Li (19 months) • Moshmi Bhagat (16 months) • Niamh Thomson (11 months) • Oliver Belmore (2 years) • Oscar Brennan (10 months) • Otto Salamon (7 months) • Otto White (12 months) • Rafael Belmas (18 months) • Reuben Nash (7 months) • Rhys MacQueen (13 months) • Ruadhán Taylor (10 months) • Ruben Brown (6 months) • Rupert Gillett (18 months) • Sam English (2 years) • Samarth Dhawan (11 months) • Scarlett Hall (10 months) • Sienna Johal (5 years) • Taliesin Swift (9 months) • Una Gormley (16 months) • Zachary Glennie (8 months) • Zane Steinberg (10 months).

And to the mums, dads + grandparents who let us take photos of them, too:

Anna-Louise Lee • Becky Kernutt • Bernadette Ward • Danielle Brown • Donna Clarke • Ellie Wetz • Gemma Moore • Grace Vincent • Jason Morrison • Karen Kooyman • Leona Melius • Manjinder Johal • Michelle Moka • Moji Ade-Onojobi • Patsy Morse • Samantha Dhanilall.

For all the advice in 'Our friends say...', thank you to the following parents + their inspirational little ones:

Angie Turner (Reece + Summer) • Belinda Middleton (Isaac + William) • Bethany Clinton (Sebastian + Jude) • Caitlin Wales (Isla) • Hannah Llywelyn-Davies (Sion + Florence) • Jo Matthews (Samuel + Evie) • Kaela Moore (Cayden) • Katie Green (Lucie) • Katrina Minoletti (Toby) • Kirsten Shepherd (Jessica) • Lottie Ainsworth-Moore (Tabitha) • Megan Sawyers (Rose) • Melanie Almenhali (Mariam, Assia + Ryan) • Natasha Tenpow (Charlie) • Nicole Borbely (Cameron + Oliver) • Nicole McDonnell (Callum + Harrison) • Pamela Newby (Paige) • Photini Konnarides (Danny + Aurelia) • Rhiannon Patel (Fox) • Sophie Harper (Tristan + Alice) • Vicki Cullen (Tilly).

For letting us take photos at their homes, and for all of the other important stuff we needed for our *First Foods* Book:

Alissa Manners, Angie Turner, Anita Mangan, Celia Huxtable, Claire Baseley, Emily Quah, Eve + Andy Pallent, Fredderick Karabela, Judy Barratt, Lincoln Jefferson, Manisha Patel, Natasha Field, Rosie Reynolds, Sam Burges, Sarah Ford, Sophie Bristow Symonds, Val Mote + Victoria Cripps.